HEAL YOUR HIPS

Also by Robert Klapper, MD, and Lynda Huey

Heal Your Knees: How to Prevent Knee Surgery & What to Do If You Need It

Also by Lynda Huey

The Complete Waterpower Workout Book (with Robert Forster, PT)
The Waterpower Workout (with R. R. Knudson)
A Running Start: An Athlete, A Woman

SECOND EDITION

HEAL YOUR HIPS

*How to Prevent Hip Surgery
and What to Do If You Need It*

**Robert Klapper, MD
and
Lynda Huey**

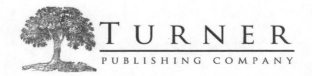

TURNER
PUBLISHING COMPANY

Turner Publishing Company
4507 Charlotte Avenue • Suite 100 • Nashville, Tennessee 37209
www.turnerpublishing.com

Heal Your Hips How to Prevent Surgery and What to Do If You Need It

Cover design: Maddie Cothren
Book design: Mallory Perkins

The information contained in this book is not intended to serve as a replacement for professional medical advice. Any use of the information in this book is at the reader's discretion. The author and the publisher specifically disclaim any and all liability arising directly or indirectly from the use or application of any information contained in this book. A health-care professional should be consulted regarding your specific situation.

The information contained in this book is not intended to be prescriptive. Any attempt to diagnose, treat, or rehabilitate an injury or disorder should come under the direction of a doctor, an orthopedic specialist, or a physical therapist. Before starting the exercises in this book, check with your doctor. Not all exercises are suitable for everyone. Anyone using these programs assumes the risk of injury from performing the exercises and/or using the equipment shown.

Library of Congress Cataloging-in-Publication Data:

Klapper, Robert.
 Heal your hips : how to prevent hip surgery and what to do if you need it / Robert Klapper, MD and Lynda Huey. -- Second edition.
    pages cm
 Includes index.
 ISBN 978-1-63026-756-8 (pbk.) -- ISBN 978-1-68162-094-7 (hardback)
 1. Hip joint--Popular works. 2. Hip joint--Surgery--Popular works. I. Huey, Lynda. II. Title.
 RD772.K53 2015
 617.5'810592--dc23
                          2015031163

Printed in the United States of America.

15 14 13 12 11 10 9 8 7 6

In memory of my father the carpenter, Abraham Klapper, and my mother the nurse, Lillian Klapper; and to my wife, Ellen Klapper, MD, and my daughter, Michele Klapper.

—Robert Klapper, MD

In memory of my father, Robert Huey; and for my mother, Glenn Margaret Huey, the angel of my life.

—Lynda Huey

CONTENTS

PREFACE

The secret of how to prevent hip surgery is now in your hands.

We needed to write a second edition of *Heal Your Hips* because there is so much new information that we wanted to share with you. The entire landscape of how we view and treat hips has changed dramatically since *Heal Your Hips* was first published in 1999. This new book on hips will bring you the updated details as well as information about the latest orthopedic breakthroughs that weren't even on our radar back then.

In 2003, a doctor in Switzerland coined the phrase FAI (femoroacetabular impingement), and this has become the hottest topic in orthopedics today. Although we mentioned labral tears in our first book, that subject has greatly expanded and is closely connected with FAI. We were the pioneers in offering the lay public an alternative to total hip surgery if they were candidates for hip arthroscopy. Today, arthroscopic hip surgeries now flourish for an entire "middle ground" of hip problems: FAI and torn labrums. And we hope that early detection of FAI and arthroscopic correction of the bony anatomy may prevent the need for hip implant surgery later in life.

What hasn't changed, however, is our original mission statement. We still wanted to convert what we both do every day into something you can walk away with, which is now in your hands. As you read this book, we want you to feel as if you've come into an examining room with me and entered a pool with Lynda Huey, and that the experience gives you a strong sense of certainty that we are going to help you get through whatever hip condition you might have.

People have told us that between my analogies and metaphors and Lynda's clear, concise writing, we are able to help our readers see pictures with our words. They have said that we make difficult orthopedic concepts easily understood, and we do it better than anyone else. We've become the team you can trust. We are your second opinion.

When we wrote the first hip book, the Internet barely existed. What we have seen is an explosion of information and a shrinking of the world. I have seen thousands of patients since that book came out, many of whom read the book, got on an airplane, and came to see me in my office and came to see Lynda Huey in her pool. It was always interesting to me to hear things like this from my patients: "I'm a skeptical person and I didn't believe how miraculous the water exercises could be in truly changing my life." The patients either prevented surgery with the pool program, or, if it turned out they had to have surgery, they had regained muscle strength and joint flexibility so that the surgery was much easier to go through.

I think our first book was so successful because we didn't just write a book. We held our readers' hands as we explained difficult concepts and helped them understand what was happening to their hips.

Now, in this new book, we're taking it to the next level with KlapperVision®. You won't find another book that uses the visual of an orange cut in half to describe the normal angle of the hip socket, but that's KlapperVision. The verbal animation of KlapperVision combines my love of art and medicine as I teach. I relish the opportunity I have on the radio with ESPN, on television with Fox Sports, and in this book to explain intricate, scientific matters in understandable ways by using household and daily-life images and relating them to the anatomical structures we discuss. That's my legacy.

I had many wild ideas in 1999 that I envisioned for the future. We included text boxes in our first book that featured stem cell and other injections into joints, as well as genetic engineering. Those things have come to pass and we discuss them in this second book. Many of these treatments are still in their infancy of research. I thought space-age technology would not exist in my lifetime, but now it's clear that this futuristic medicine is going to be here soon. So in this new book we will once again look at where I think the future of medicine will go next. Add what we know now to the new treatments to come, and we may make the need for artificial joints obsolete.

And yet Lynda and I have our feet firmly rooted in basic knowledge: I as a marble stone carver and Lynda as the authority on water rehabilitation. It doesn't get more basic on planet Earth than rock and water. Lynda grasps the body as a complex machine that must move in order to heal well. My expertise is below the skin. I have done about five hundred surgeries a year over the past twenty-five years. I have learned so much from my patients that my own truths have developed, and I no longer merely accept the dogma I learned in medical school. At the time of this writing, I have opened up over twelve thousand people for surgery. The sheer magnitude of that number allows me to take a history from a patient, do a physical exam, look at his or her studies (X-rays, MRIs, CT scans), and as I touch the patient's skin, I am literally able to see through it to the anatomy that lies below. Many a student or resident who has come to operate with me has asked, "Dr. Klapper, why did you put your surgical instrument here and not there?" My response is, "Because I know that the artery and the nerve are behind that bone." And they say, "I don't see that." And I say, "Someday you will."

In a similar way, Lynda has developed her keen coach's eye over the past decades. She will say to a patient, "You don't see the muscle tone coming in yet, but I can see it. I know where your muscles and your hip are going to be a month from now. I know what strength you will have and what you will be capable of doing. There's no magic. All you have to do is show up and do the work."

Imagine having that sixth sense about the body. That's where we both are today. We know so much more now than when we wrote our first book because we learn from our patients every day. That's what we want to share with you.

This is what makes the Revised and Updated Second Edition so exciting!

—Robert Klapper, MD
Beverly Hills, California

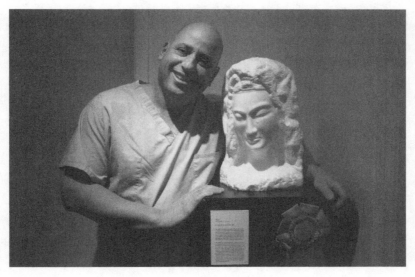

Dr. Klapper with his prize-winning sculpture, "Pieta." He sculpts in Carrara, Italy, using the same stone and the same chisel as Michelangelo.

Dr. Klapper and I met in 1993 right after he performed Wilt Chamberlain's hip arthroscopy. Wilt had heard from one of the volleyball players at Muscle Beach in Santa Monica that Dr. Klapper had scoped his hip. Wilt's hip had been bothering him for years, and the small scope surgery sounded a lot better to him than a total hip replacement.

Wilt raced over to meet Dr. Klapper, and the two of them hit it off immediately. Wilt told Dr. Klapper how I had helped him rehab his knee and elbow in water, and he must have bragged about me because Dr. Klapper wanted to meet me right away. It was clear when I met him that he was serious about wanting to help his patients prevent hip surgery. Dr. Klapper could tell I was serious about helping my clients and patients of all levels seek physical excellence. As we talked, I learned from his point of view why my pool program was successful: if patients regained strength and flexibility in the muscles surrounding their hips, they could become pain-free without surgery. It simply wouldn't matter what their X-rays or MRIs looked like if they were able to function well in daily life.

Before long, Dr. Klapper was sending dozens of patients into my pool. He invited me into his operating room to observe him at work. I watched over his shoulder while in a single morning he gave several patients new, well-functioning hips.

Early in my water rehab career, I learned a lot from working with Olympic sprinters, jumpers, and hurdlers, and from professional basketball, ice hockey, tennis, and football players. Because of my own previous athletic career, I understood their urgency to keep training and to return to their sport. I found ways to keep them working out after any injury. "There's always something we can do in the pool," I would tell them. The athletes, their coaches, and I saw that not only could we keep elite athletes in great shape while their injuries healed but that our efforts in the pool also speeded the healing of injuries. Some of these athletes ran personal best times their first day out of the pool. In fact, one woman actually won an Olympic gold medal right after we trained a month in the pool. We knew we were on to something!

That "something" has evolved over the years into pool programs so that people of all fitness levels can make physical improvements in the water. We modified the high-speed running, jumping, and kicking exercises to slower speeds with less amplitude and force. It turned out that even the gentlest of movements in water created resistance to build strength; even the slowest deep-water interval training enhanced aerobic fitness; and even the most deliberate and careful walking across the pool helped improve balance.

Hundreds of doctors refer patients to my pool program every year. We take pride in offering the gold standard in pool therapy combined with traditional land therapy. All of our patients get to rehab like world-class athletes, aiming at high goals. People at every step along the movement continuum—from those in wheelchairs who can barely move, to those with various aches and pains, to patients recovering from orthopedic surgeries, to professional and Olympic athletes—are all encouraged to seek excellence, whatever the definition of excellence might be for their conditions.

People often ask for my criteria of a good pool-therapy program. Here it is. The pool water is between 87 and 92 degrees. Bars are on the sides of the pool for bracing, kicking, stretching, and tethering. Half the pool is deep water and the other half is shallow water. Deep water is where we gain more than half the healing benefit by exercising without the feet touching the pool bottom. Therapists are in the water next to the patients, not standing or squatting on the deck. Pool work is hands-on work, so therapists are close enough to patients to give manual cues with their hands or feet and to adjust the body position of someone struggling to find good form. The exercises are based on the buoyancy and resistance of water, unlike land exercises, which are based on gravity.

Dr. Klapper and I receive emails from people around the world seeking guidance with their hip problems. We answer all of those emails, and we have found that there are few pool programs that meet the above criteria. So we began this new book to share our concepts with as many hip patients as possible. We intend to write many more books together, and I have launched my Aquatic Rehab Online Course so anyone can learn the pool program anywhere in the world straight from a computer or mobile device.

From my point of view, it would be hard to match Dr. Klapper's insight, experience, and charisma, so I completely understand why you would want to fly to Los Angeles to see him. You could also come to my pool to learn an individualized pool program to serve you and your hip for the rest of your life. But if you can't get to Los Angeles, we want this second edition of *Heal Your Hips* to provide you with the knowledge and skills to make it through the challenge you're facing with your hip.

Keep reading to learn how to reduce or eliminate your hip pain, which will allow you to become active again. Our exercise programs have been astonishingly successful, sparing many of our patients the surgical procedures described later in the book.

Flip through the book, get excited about regaining your mobility, and commit today to the self-help that follows.

—Lynda Huey
Santa Monica, California

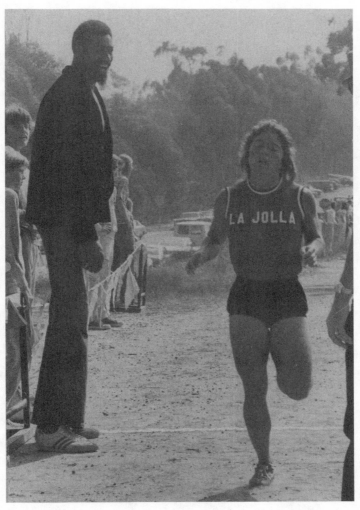

Lynda Huey with Wilt Chamberlain, watching her cross the finish line in 1974. Lynda's own injuries led her into the water to create healing programs for athletes, which became her life's work—aquatic rehabilitation.

ACKNOWLEDGMENTS

The following people contributed to the success of this book:

Orthopedic surgeon Jason Snibbe, MD, contributed the material in chapter 13 and allowed Lynda Huey and Ashley White, DPT, to observe several hip arthroscopy surgeries. He was generous with his time in helping plan the protocols in chapter 16 for post-surgical hip arthroscopy patients.

Radiologist Douglas Brown, MD, provided new studies in chapter 4 and educated Lynda Huey on the latest developments in MR arthrograms as well as the two newest findings: an alpha angle on an MRI and a crossover sign on an X-ray.

Ashley White, DPT, contributed the land exercises in chapters 1 and 12, and she eloquently explained how the combination of pool and land exercises work magically together—how using the two together produces a better result than either one alone. She added new material to chapters 11 and 16, and she participated in the land exercise photo shoot.

Jennifer Cabrera, PA, Dr. Snibbe's physician assistant, worked tirelessly to help us find photos for chapter 13. She facilitated access to the operating room for Lynda Huey and Ashley White, DPT, to observe surgeries with Dr. Snibbe.

Naomi Tashman, RN, BSN, ONC, WCC, a nurse on the orthopedic unit at Cedars-Sinai Medical Center, significantly contributed her clinical expertise to chapter 15.

James Cowan took over the day-to-day operations of CompletePT so Lynda could devote her time to the writing of this book. His quiet presence made it possible for Lynda to have solitude and yet immediate technical support in managing the documents and photos. He posed for photos with Dr. Klapper in chapter 3, in the biking shot in chapter 7, and in the movement precautions in chapter 15. He was the invaluable strength and smarts behind our ability to put together so many gorgeous photos. His creativity in shooting the oranges brought life to that KlapperVision sequence in chapter 4. He shot the photo of Dr. Klapper and his sculpture in the preface, and he provided the necessary touch-ups and modifications on photos, drawings, charts, and figures.

Anesthesiologist Matthew R. Eng, MD, offered well-written input on the use of anesthesia in chapter 15. He and anesthesiologist Kapil Anand, MD, make surgery as painless as possible for Dr. Klapper's patients.

LaReine Chabut once again made it easy to shoot our exercise photos, both pool and land. She graces the cover, and she also contributed material about Pilates exercises in chapter 6.

Jessica Bufete, DPT, reviewed chapter 16 and added new, well-written material to it.

Lora Fremont graciously allowed us to use her pool for the photo shoots.

Rod Klein shot dazzling pool photos for us.

Robert Reiff shot the beautiful land photos.

Marjorie Kaye did the medical illustrations in chapters 2 and 3.

LeRoy Perry Jr., DC, a pioneer in sports medicine and aquatic therapy, guided Lynda Huey into the water and provided a solid base of support for her physical therapy business, CompletePT Pool & Land Physical Therapy.

Mark Frantz, Dr. Klapper's X-ray technician, gathered X-rays for chapter 4.

Bibi Vabrey, Dr. Klapper's office manager, contributed the material in chapter 3 on forming positive relationships with the doctor's staff.

Adriana Iturrios, Adelle Baumgard, Marion Dillon, Yvette Velazquez, Susan Chavez, and physician assistant Katie Pavlisko in Dr. Klapper's office, all lent their invaluable support whenever needed.

Orthopedic technician Gene Crawford has the wisest hands in helping Dr. Klapper do his surgeries.

Donna Aiello, head operating room nurse, makes sure every day in the operating room is a magical experience for Dr. Klapper.

Gigi Guest, Lynda's personal assistant, held everything together during the long months of Lynda Huey's book-writing seclusion.

Jane Hasle, Lynda's COO at CompletePT, used her keen reading skills to catch typos and offer improvements to the manuscript. She served as an invaluable sounding board to Lynda Huey as they did final edits of the manuscript.

Daniel Lim, MD, contributed material to chapter 5. He is the youngest contributor and represents the future of the field of orthopedics.

Dustin Burkes did the drawings in chapters 5 and 13.

XVIII ACKNOWLEDGMENTS

Leslie Kaminoff updated the yoga material in chapter 6.

Mike Shapow, PT, contributed material to chapter 11.

Literary agents Danielle Egan-Miller and Abby Saul assisted in bringing this book to fruition.

Zan Knudson helped write the first edition of this book and, even though she's gone, she silently coached Lynda Huey through the writing process of this second edition.

Jonathan Segal launched Lynda Huey's writing career and was her first editor at Quadrangle/New York Times Book Co. In retrospect, his patience and kindness were staggering. He conceived the title of Lynda's book, *A Running Start: An Athlete, A Woman*, which forty years later is back in print in paperback.

1

THE MAGIC OF WATER AND MOVEMENT

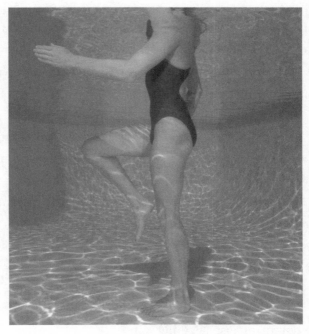

Photo 1-2. Marching.

Your hip hurts, and you don't know what to do about it.

We're here to help: an orthopedic surgeon who tries to keep his patients out of the operating room and a water rehab specialist whose pool program is followed worldwide. Together we help guide our patients to their own solutions by educating them. Since you have this book, you're ready to get started.

We want you to become a better patient by learning more about the condition of your hip. When your doctor asks you, "Where does it hurt?" we want you to be able to give clear information. You'll learn to tell your physical history well, which is incredibly important in finding the right diagnosis. We want you to know what questions to ask and where to find answers. You will become a well-educated patient who feels empowered to walk through what can feel like a medical labyrinth. Along the way you'll learn potential reasons for your pain, you'll discover basic concepts about X-rays and MRIs, and you'll look at a vast array of possible treatments that can help reduce your pain. Keep reading. It's time to start gathering the data you'll need as you seek an answer for your hip.

Let's say you've just come home from a long walk or bike ride and suddenly discover a deep ache in your hip. Or maybe your hip has been bothering you off and on for weeks. The pain keeps you awake at night. You're even starting to limp. Perhaps you were told years ago that you have a "hip condition" that was bound to be troublesome later in life. Now you fear your pain will go on forever.

Whether your hip pain is a surprise or a problem you've been expecting, you want relief. In our experience, starting to move in water can be the best possible thing you can do for immediate pain reduction. So that's what we'll do first.

Go to your nearest swimming pool and do the fifteen-minute program that follows. The pain relief will be worth the effort of traveling to the water.

Fifteen-Minute Pool Program

You don't need any equipment, just a bathing suit.

Make a photocopy of the shaded box on page 3 and laminate it to take to the pool with you. Place it poolside and follow the order of the exercises. Do each exercise for about one minute.

While doing the exercises, focus on the physical abilities of your affected and unaffected hips. Notice whether you take a longer stride with one leg than with the other or whether you can lift one leg higher to the side. Pay attention to when and where your hip hurts. Does it hurt in the groin as you lift your leg to the side? Does it hurt on the side of your hip as you cross your legs? Start gathering information.

Fifteen-Minute Pool Program

Exercise 1. Walking Forward, Backward,
Sideways

Exercise 2. Marching

Exercise 3. Bicycling

Exercise 4. Scissors

Exercise 5. Lateral Leg Raises

Exercise 6. Leg Swings

Exercise 7. Knee Swivels

Exercise 8. Squats

Exercise 9. Hamstring Stretch

Exercise 10. Lateral Split

Exercise 1. Shallow Water Walking Warm-up

Spend at least three of your fifteen minutes on this exercise—one minute forward, one backward, and one sideways. Do all the forward walking, then all the backward, turning each time you cross the pool. Most pools are slanted at least a little, so by turning, you'll alternate which of your legs is on the uphill and which is on the downhill. That helps even out the stress placed on your sore hip. Within a few minutes, you will have become accustomed to the water temperature. Now face the deep end of the pool and walk sideways without turning around so that you lead alternately with the weaker hip and stronger hip each time you cross the pool.

Exercise 2. Marching

Begin marching by lifting one of your knees as high as you can without hip discomfort or pain. If you encounter pain, lower your knee. Lean forward and take a step, then lift the other knee to a similar position. Pay attention to the direction your knees are pointing while you march. Use bent arms in opposition to the bent knees. Move your right arm in time with your left knee, and your left arm with your right knee. You don't need to lift your knee as high as in Photo 1-2 on page 1. This is a goal to strive for, but it may not be where you begin.

Exercise 3. Bicycling

Brace yourself at the side of the pool or sit on a step. Bend your knees to begin kicking in a bicycling movement as shown in Photo 1-3.

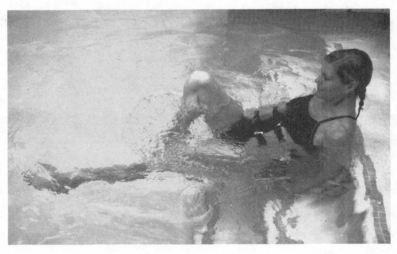

Photo 1-3. Bicycling.

If crossing your legs hurts, simply open your legs wide, then close your legs until your ankles touch.

Sit on a step to do this exercise or push your lower back against the side of the pool to brace yourself. Lift both legs up and open them wide apart as shown in Photo 1-4A. Then with a scissors motion, cross one leg over the top of the other as in Photo 1-4B. Continue crossing and opening them, alternating the top leg. Use as much force in opening the legs as you use in crossing them. Make sure your knees point upward, not outward.

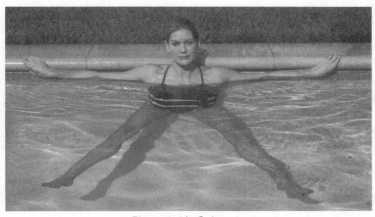

Photo 1-4A. Scissors.

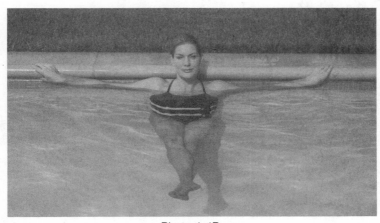

Photo 1-4B.

Exercise 5. Lateral Leg Raises

Stand with your hand on the side of the pool, facing the end of the pool as in Photo 1-5A. Lift your leg directly to the side as high as you comfortably can without changing your erect posture. (See Photo 1-5B.) Don't lean to the side in order to lift your leg higher. Keep the feet parallel so that your knee and foot point forward rather than upward. Pull your leg back to the starting position. Apply equal force as you lift the leg up and pull it down.

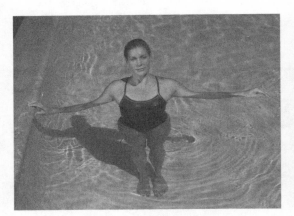

Photo 1-5A. Lateral Leg Raises.

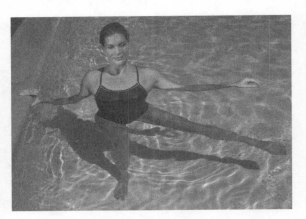

Photo 1-5B.

Listen to Your Body

As you position yourself for these exercises, you might feel the urge to move your leg or body in a way that isn't part of the program. That's your body talking to you: do what it tells you. For example, if you feel like pulling your knee toward your chest to loosen your back and buttocks, do it. Intuitive knowledge surfaces in the water, so pay attention to what you're feeling and what movements your body asks of you.

—Lynda Huey

If you have lower back problems, don't swing your leg so far behind you. If you feel hip pain as you reach your leg forward, don't lift it so high. If you have **hip flexor tendinitis** *or have a torn labrum, reach only slightly to the front and emphasize the backward swing.*

Stand erect with your hand on the side of the pool for stability. Swing your leg straight forward as shown in Photo 1-6A, then swing it down and to the rear as shown in Photo 1-6B. If a full swing forward hurts your hip, don't lift it so high. If a full swing backward hurts your back, don't reach so far. After thirty seconds, turn and perform leg swings with the other leg.

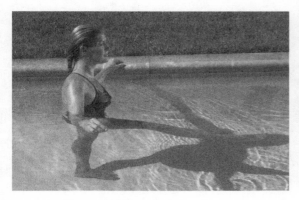
Photo 1-6A. Leg Swings.

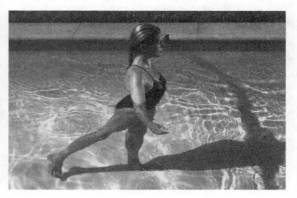
Photo 1-6B.

Stand on your left leg with your right knee bent as in Photo 1-7A. Your right hip and knee are both bent to 90 degrees throughout the exercise. For stability, tighten the muscles of your left leg and buttock. Do not allow any movement at the standing hip; all movement comes strictly from the working hip. Swivel your right knee outward to reach the position shown in Photo 1-7B, then return to the starting position or even farther across the body if you can do so without pain. Keep your foot directly beneath your knee. Reach as far as you can in each direction. After thirty seconds, turn and repeat with the other leg. Notice if this is easier to do with one leg than the other.

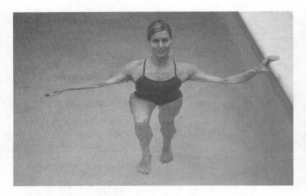

Photo 1-7A. Knee Swivels.   Photo 1-7B.

Water Works!

Here's how water works: As soon as you step into the pool, you've eliminated the weight-bearing part of your problem. Once you've taken a "load" off your painful hip, you move it through its range of motion against the smooth, three-dimensional resistance of the water. Your hip gets stronger. Water is like a strategic missile that knows its target and continues to pursue it. No matter how you move in water, it works to strengthen the muscles surrounding your hip joint.

Exercise 8. Squats

Face the side of the pool in chest-deep water with your feet parallel and shoulder-width apart as in Photo 1-8A. Grasp the edge of the pool with both hands. Keep your back straight and slowly bend both knees until you've lowered your chin to the water as shown in Photo 1-8B. Your heels will probably lift away from the pool bottom. If they do, push them down as you stand to the starting position.

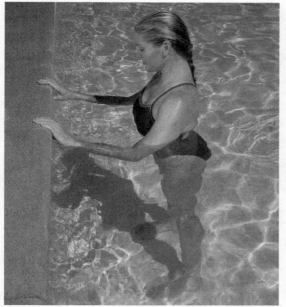

Photo 1-8A. Squats.

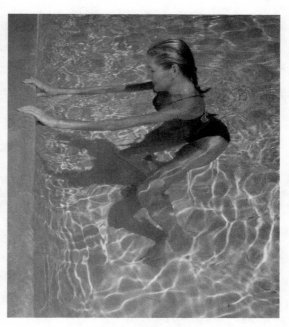

Photo 1-8B.

Exercise 9. Hamstring Stretch

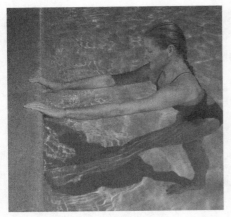

Photo 1-9. Hamstring Stretch.

Grasp the side of the pool with both hands. Place your left foot, toes up, against the pool wall as shown in Photo 1-9. Keep your neck, shoulders, arms, and back relaxed throughout the exercise. Gently straighten your left knee as far as you can while you breathe deeply and slowly. If this causes too much pain, lower your foot on the pool wall until you can comfortably do this stretch. Repeat with the other leg.

Exercise 10. Lateral Split

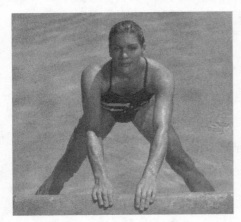

Photo 1-10. Lateral Split.

Continue grasping the side of the pool. Place both feet, toes up, against the pool wall as shown in Photo 1-10. Gradually walk your feet apart, opening your legs to the side as far as you comfortably can. To take pressure off your ankles and knees, let your feet turn out slightly. Breathe slowly and deeply at least five times as you hold this stretch.

You'll probably discover that you don't want to get out of the pool after only fifteen minutes. It feels so good, you'll want to return day after day. In that case, turn to chapters 8 and 9 to get ready for a full pool program. Choose a flotation belt right away so you can experience the miraculous feeling of exercising your sore hip without any weight on it at all. See page 117 for flotation belts. If you have already had hip surgery, you will start with chapter 10 on page 173.

Fifteen-Minute Land Program

When you return from the pool, find a carpeted area, or use a comfortable yoga mat on a hardwood floor for these exercises. You will need a towel for Exercises 13 and 15. We've allocated about two minutes to each exercise. Begin each exercise by moving or stretching your unaffected side first. In that way, you will learn what is normal for you and be able to compare it to the affected side later. If an exercise or stretch causes pain, skip it for now so that you don't increase your symptoms. You can try it again next week.

Exercise 11. Knee to Chest Stretch

Lie on your back with your legs straight. Keep your head and lower back flat on the floor throughout this stretch. Pull the knee of your unaffected leg toward your chest as in Photo 1-11. If you feel pain, release the stretch slightly to a position that is comfortable. Your affected leg remains flat on the floor unless you feel pain, in which case you can bend it slightly. Hold this stretch while you breathe deeply and slowly at least five times. Consciously relax with every exhalation. Come back to the starting position, then perform the stretch slowly on your affected side. As you breathe deeply, you may be surprised to feel that your affected hip allows a bit more movement with each breath. Repeat on each side.

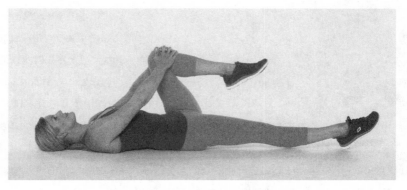

Photo 1-11. Knee to Chest Stretch.

Exercise 12. Hip Extensor Stretch

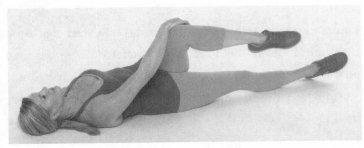

Photo 1-12. Hip Extensor Stretch.

Continue lying on your back. Use your hand to pull the knee of your unaffected leg toward your opposite shoulder until you feel a stretch in the buttocks. If you feel any pain or pinching in the front of that hip, release the stretch slightly. Let your affected leg lie flat on the floor, or you can bend the knee slightly if you feel pain. Hold this stretch while you breathe deeply and slowly at least five times. Consciously relax with every exhalation. Return to the starting position, then perform the stretch slowly on your affected side. Repeat on each side.

Exercise 13. Hamstring Stretch

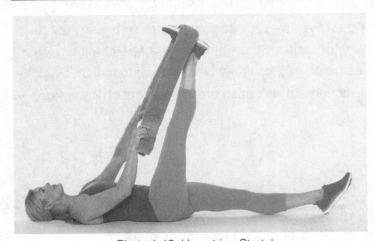

Photo 1-13. Hamstring Stretch.

Although this stretch was already done in the pool, it needs to be done on land too. If you have a back condition, keep one knee bent with your foot on the floor while you raise the other leg. Start with your unaffected leg. Lie on your back with a towel or strap around the ball of your foot. Slowly lift your unaffected leg toward the ceiling and straighten your knee until you feel a stretch along the back of your thigh and knee as in Photo 1-13. Keep your knee as straight as possible. Hold the stretch while you breathe slowly and deeply at least five times. When you feel the muscles relax, first try to straighten the knee more fully, then gently lift your leg higher. Now perform the stretch slowly on your affected leg. Repeat on each side.

Exercise 14. Bridge

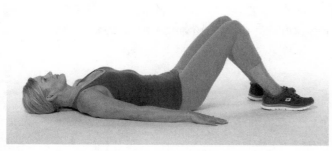

Photo 1-14A. Bridge.

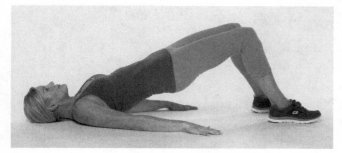

Photo 1-14B.

Bend your knees and place your feet flat on the floor with your arms straight down at your sides as in Photo 1-14A. Allow your back to rest in its natural position and contract your abdominal muscles. Lift your buttocks off the floor to the position shown in Photo 1-14B and hold for five seconds before returning to the starting position. Do ten reps.

Exercise 15. Prone Hip Extension

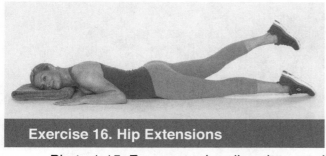

Exercise 16. Hip Extensions

Assume a face down (prone) position with your head turned to the side. Contract your buttocks and abdominal muscles to stabilize your torso. Keep your knees straight and slowly raise your unaffected leg off the floor as in Photo 1-15. Focus on primarily using your buttocks muscles. Hold the leg up for two seconds, then slowly return it to the floor. Do this ten times, then repeat on the affected side. You can turn your head to the opposite side any time you wish.

Photo 1-15. Prone Hip Extension.

Assume a balanced position on your hands and knees as in Photo 1-16A. Lift your unaffected leg out behind you until your leg is parallel with the floor as in Photo 1-16B. Return to the starting position on your hands and knees. Do ten repetitions on each side.

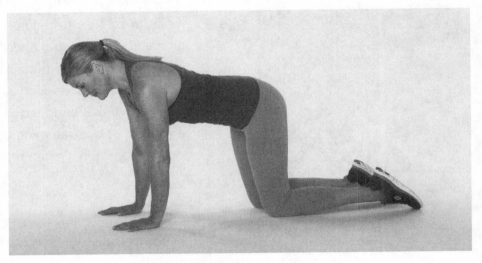

Photo 1-16A. Hip Extensions.

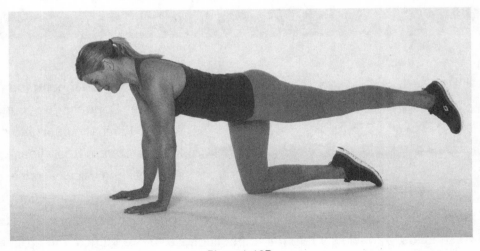

Photo 1-16B.

Exercise 17. Single Leg Balance

HEAL YOUR HIPS

Stand in front of a chair, counter, or solid surface that you can hold for balance. Find a focal point, stand erect, and tighten your abdominals and buttocks. Let go of the chair. Once you feel stable, lift your affected leg just slightly, which will force you to balance on the unaffected leg as in Photo 1-17. Stand for fifteen seconds or until you lose your balance and need to hold on to the counter or solid surface. Perform the same exercise while standing on the affected leg. Repeat on each side. Each day that you do this exercise, try to add at least one second to your balancing time. Make thirty seconds your goal and work your way up to that.

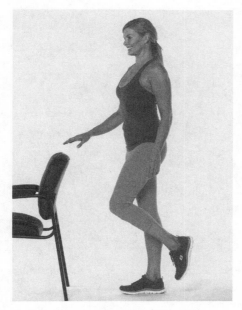

Photo 1-17. Single Leg Balance.

After your fifteen minutes in water and fifteen minutes on land, you will probably feel your hip moving more smoothly and with a greater sense of ease. You have discovered some important truths:

• Water exercise allows you to perform movements that would be painful to do on land.
• Land exercise more closely duplicates the challenges you must face in daily life.
• Movement heals.

2

HIP BASICS

Go to your freezer and take out two ice cubes. Wet them and rub them against each other. Feel how slippery they are. There is almost no friction as one glides across the surface of the other.

Next, consider a healthy hip joint. The two surfaces of that joint are even more slippery than the ice cubes. As the hip bends, rotates, and straightens, the contact between the two halves of the joint is so delicate that the friction is less than that of your two ice cubes.

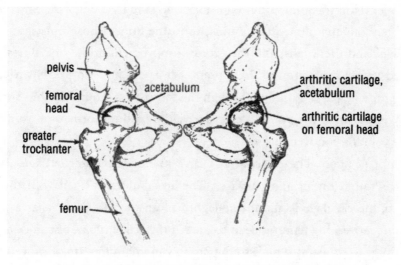

Drawing 2-1. Left, healthy hip joint; right, osteoarthritis.

The hip is where the femur (thigh bone) attaches to the pelvis in a ball-and-socket joint. (See Drawing 2-1.) The upper end of the femur is shaped like a ball and forms the femoral head. That head rotates in a socket called the acetabulum, which is formed by the pelvic bones. The hip joint is extremely strong, and at the same time it is durable and offers great range of movement.

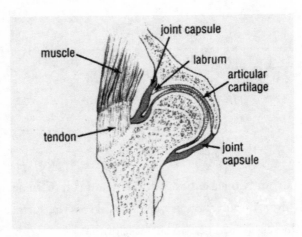

Drawing 2-2. Hip joint capsule with surrounding soft tissues.

The tough fibers and ligaments that encase the hip joint are called the joint capsule. These connective tissues envelop the joint and hold it together. (See Drawing 2-2.) Surrounding the joint are muscles and tendons that attach those muscles to the bone. Those muscles are located in the buttocks, the pelvis, and the thighs, and they control movement at the hip. Bursal sacs filled with fluids are situated in key spots around the hip and act as cushions to prevent friction and relieve pressure between moving parts. Running through the soft tissues around the hip are various sensory nerves that carry impulses to the brain to create sensation and motor nerves from the brain to the muscles to create voluntary movement.

In a healthy hip, the femoral head is covered with a layer of **articular cartilage**, also called **hyaline cartilage**, which is found on all joint surfaces. The acetabulum is lined with this same articular cartilage. In a hip, the cartilage is about one-eighth of an inch thick and has a firm consistency. When the hip joint moves, the femoral head rotates in the acetabulum, but since articular cartilage has no nerve endings to transmit signals to the brain, you are not aware of movement between the two cartilage layers, and you don't feel any friction. Nor do you feel the constant trauma of weight bearing when you walk, run, or do any of your other physical activities. This miraculous cartilage that provides such elegance is like your permanent teeth: you get only one set.

Articular cartilage does not have a blood supply. Rather, it receives its nourishment from a flow of fluids. Here's a KlapperVision: Picture a spongy mop soaking up water and then being rung out again. When the joint is at rest, the spongy material that comprises cartilage soaks up liquid, which is

HEAL YOUR HIPS

synovial fluid. Then, when you put pressure on that hip joint by taking a step, it squeezes the fluid out again. When you lift your leg to take another step, the fluid rushes back into the cartilage. The fluid moves in and out as your cartilage responds to the changing forces exerted on your hip joint. This process both nourishes and lubricates the cartilage cells.

Where Does Your Hip Hurt?

When patients come to see me and say their hip hurts, they usually point to one of three places:

1. The front. They point to their groin and think they have a hernia. They often also have pain that goes down the front of their thigh, but it stops at the knee. This is a classic indicator that we need to investigate the ball-and-socket joint. It could be arthritis, a labral tear, or a torn muscle.

2. The side. Patients point to their hip pocket and say it hurts right there. This is the classic indication of **bursitis**. Yes, you can have bursitis-type pain on the side of your hip because your hip joint is deteriorating. But you can also have a perfectly normal ball-and-socket joint and just have inflammation of the muscles and the bursal sac. Point tenderness on a specific spot on the side of your hip is the classic indicator for bursitis.

3. The back. Patients will make a fist and punch their buttock, saying their hip hurts right there. What they're generally pointing to is the **sacroiliac joint**. The patient will think they have hip pain when in fact that location leads either to their pelvis or their spine, not the hip joint.

—Robert Klapper, MD

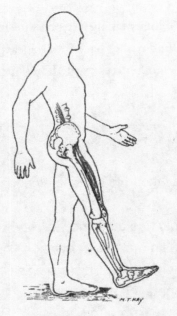

Drawing 2-3. Hip flexors.

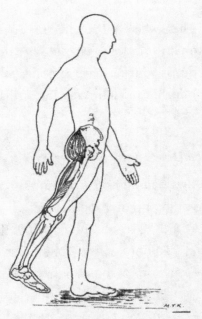

Drawing 2-4. Hip extensors.

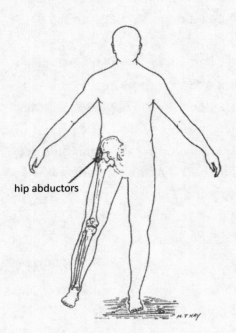

hip abductors

Drawing 2-5. Hip abductors.

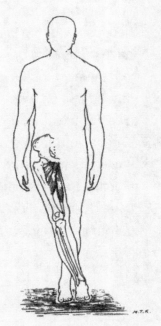

Drawing 2-6. Hip adductors.

The Muscles That Move the Hip

Muscles work in synchronized pairs: when one contracts, the opposing one relaxes. The muscles executing the actual movement are known as **agonists**. As the agonists contract, the opposing muscle group, the **antagonists**, must relax to allow movement to occur. For example, when you lift your leg forward, the hip flexors serve as the agonists to initiate the movement, while the opposing hip extensors, the antagonists, relax to allow movement to occur. Conversely, if you reach your leg backward, the muscles reverse roles: the extensors are the agonists, while the flexors are the antagonists.

The muscle pairs of the hip are the flexors/extensors (Drawings 2-3 and 2-4 on page 20), abductors/adductors (Drawings 2-5 and 2-6 on page 20), and internal rotators/external rotators. External and internal rotators combine the muscles shown in all the drawings to turn the knee and foot outward (external rotators) or inward (internal rotators).

The Negative Spiral: Loss of Hip Function

Once you start to feel pain or limited movement in your hip, a downward spiral begins. If you've been aware of your pain for a while but have taken no measures to combat your hip condition, you may have already entered this Negative Spiral. First you feel pain or limitation of movement, so you move your hip less often. You stop running, bicycling, and working out in the gym.

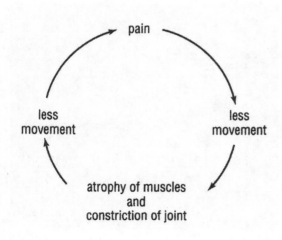

Figure 2-1. Negative Spiral.

You begin driving your car to places you used to walk to. As the pain continues, you may even find yourself taking a grocery cart to lean on even though only three items are on your list. Because you are moving your hip joint less, it isn't receiving the fluids and nourishment it requires, and it becomes further constricted and inflamed. The muscles begin shrinking, a process called **atrophy**. Once these muscles start feeling weak, you use them even less, and they atrophy even more. The tendons and capsule around the hip joint aren't being stretched to their usual length, and they begin to lose their elasticity. They become brittle and likely to split or break.

Here's some KlapperVision, an analogy that you can apply to your sore hip: Imagine you've broken your foot and doctors put it in a cast so the bones can heal. But the cast also confines the muscles and tendons of your calf. When the cast comes off weeks later, the X-ray looks fine, but your leg is shriveled from disuse. Now you have aches and pains coming from the tissues that were immobilized. The tendons haven't moved, so they weren't lubricated and they lost flexibility. The muscles didn't contract, so they atrophied and lost strength. In the same way, if you stop moving your hip due to pain, you are virtually placing your hip in a cast, and the muscles and tendons around your hip will suffer the same fate as those around the broken foot.

It is indeed a Negative Spiral: lack of movement causes increased soft tissue involvement, which in turn causes more pain, so you move even less.

You want to turn this cycle around, and you can. You can bring the soft tissues back to health, which eliminates the secondary aches and pains.

If you've bought this book, you probably already have pain or limited motion in your hip joint. If you nodded with recognition while reading about the Negative Spiral, you may have already decreased your activity and begun to notice that your hip is getting worse. It's time to learn more about what is going wrong with your hip.

The Main Causes of Hip Problems

The main causes of hip problems are:

- Osteoarthritis
- Labral tears
- Hip dysplasia
- Femoroacetabular impingement
- Posttraumatic osteoarthritis
- Avascular necrosis
- Soft-tissue injuries
- Rheumatoid arthritis

Osteoarthritis

Osteoarthritis is the most common cause of hip problems. It affects millions of people worldwide, including more than fifty-two million Americans. Known as the "wear-and-tear" form of arthritis, it was formerly thought to be caused by excessive stress to the joints from high-impact activities, but more recent studies tell us that regular exercise does not predispose us to osteoarthritis. In fact, appropriate, regular exercise can increase the functional capability of osteoarthritis patients.

Called OA for short, osteoarthritis appears in two distinct forms: primary and secondary. Primary OA is the most common and usually strikes the weight-bearing joints after the age of forty-five. We don't yet know the exact cause of primary OA, but obesity and family history are known to be risk factors. Secondary OA often appears before the age of forty and can usually be linked to a specific cause such as injury, the use of certain medications, or even joint infection or metabolic imbalances such as gout.

As we age, OA can dry out our crucial cartilage, deteriorating this protective cushion between the bones. As the disease progresses, the cartilage begins to grow brittle and to crack. Its surface may become pitted and uneven. There may even be "potholes" on the surface (see Drawing 2-2 on page 18). Although osteoarthritis begins in the articular cartilage and is primarily focused on the cartilage, it also affects other areas in and around the hip joint, including the muscles and tendons adjacent to the joint and the capsule surrounding the hip joint, and the ends of the bones just below the cartilage. We call that the **subchondral** bone. *Sub* means below and *chondral* refers to the cartilage.

KlapperVision: Picture your kitchen floor. Think of the cartilage as your linoleum and the subchondral bone as the wooden beams below the linoleum. If you spill milk on your floor when there's a crack in the linoleum, the milk will run through the linoleum and rot the wood that's underneath. Similarly, when the cartilage cracks, the synovial joint fluid escapes into the cells in the bone below the cartilage where it can form pockets of water, and like the milk, begin to rot what's underneath. That is the birth of **subchondral cysts**, one of the indicators of OA. You will learn more about these cysts in chapter 4.

The classic early symptom of arthritis is that you know when it's going to rain. When the barometric pressure changes quickly, you start to feel the deep, deep pain of arthritis. Other signs of arthritis specifically in the hip include pain when first standing up after sitting for a while and loss of internal rotation, which means not being able to point your toe inward.

Your body has the ability to tell you that something is not quite right. Around an arthritic joint, your body might give you a clue with tendinitis (see page 30). Mysteriously, the pain is not always in the spot where the real problem is. In the very early stages of arthritis in the hip, don't be surprised if your knee isn't feeling just right or if you're having a groin muscle ache. That can be an early tip-off that something isn't right deep in the joint nearby.

The Four Stages of Arthritis

Stage 1—scratches on the surface of your cartilage as if you'd scraped it with your fingernails.

Stage 2—deeper cracks and fissures that run vertically from the surface through the full thickness of the cartilage down to the bone.

Stage 3—exposed areas that could be called bald spots or potholes.

Stage 4—bone on bone so that your bones are changing shape as they grind into each other.

If your arthritis is Stage 2, it will most likely be called "mild." Stage 3 is called "moderate," and Stage 4 is "severe." Today's MRIs aren't yet sophisticated enough to tell the degree of the damage except on both ends of the spectrum. We can identify Stages 1 and 4.

The cracks or fissures in your cartilage are better known as **chondromalacia.** *Chondro* in Greek means cartilage, and *malacia* means softening of the tissues, so when you put them together, it means the softening of cartilage. This term can be confusing because it is often associated primarily with the knee. But in fact, it is a descriptive term about all cartilage in the body as it progresses through the stages of arthritis.

The other types of hip problems are described below. If your symptoms don't fit into any of the following categories, you probably have osteoarthritis.

Labral Tears

The **labrum** is a ring of rubbery fibrocartilage that attaches to the rim of your hip socket. It acts like a seal or gasket to hold the lubricating joint fluid inside the hip, as well as effectively deepening the socket and increasing the "capture" of the socket onto the ball. (See Figure 5-2B on page 76.) Probably

90 percent of all labral tears are a result of the **microtrauma** of impingement, where your own hip joint repeatedly pinches and tears the fibrocartilage of the labrum. But you can also tear your labrum because of **macrotrauma**, a sudden, severe impact such as in martial arts, a football game, or a car accident. Usually it is twisting forces that cause a detachment or virtual ungluing of the labrum from where it is affixed to the bony rim of the acetabulum.

In years past, we were concerned about the labrum tearing and flipping into the joint, where it could act like sandpaper and start to scratch the surface of the articular cartilage and therefore be a cause of osteoarthritis. Previously, we trimmed it out, just as surgeons used to trim out torn pieces of a meniscus in the knee. Now the thinking has changed. These days we respect the importance of the labrum and meniscus and work to save them at all costs. We reattach the labrum to the acetabular rim if it has been detached, or if it has been destroyed, we can reconstruct it with other tendon tissue from the body. Just as surgeons use a portion of your patellar tendon or hamstring tendon to create a new **ACL** graft, we have recently learned to use a piece of your **iliotibial band** from the outside of your thigh to create a new labrum.

Hip Dysplasia

Hip dysplasia is a congenital condition in which the hip socket develops abnormally over an entire lifetime. If the ball of the hip isn't inside the socket during the development of the fetus and infant, the two pieces of the hip don't have a chance to mold to each other. Without the influence of the socket to guide its development, the femoral head can become a **coxa magna**, a mushroom-shaped head, rather than smooth and round. On the socket side, what is supposed to be a nice, round dome becomes a flatter surface because the ball wasn't there to force the spherical growth. Nearly always, the deformity has led to a smaller, shallower socket. Only rarely does the deformity take the form of a larger socket than normal.

Hip dysplasia is something the hip develops from the fetal stage into early childhood, into early adulthood, and finally into adulthood. This condition has its own clock: it can cause pain and limited function at any point in life. Dysplasia is usually diagnosed early in a person's life, so you may already know if you have it. Yet some patients with hip dysplasia don't come into my office until they are in their 20s, 30s, 40s, or even 50s. Generally they have had hip pain for many years, but they never received the correct diagnosis. Their hip isn't dislocating even though the socket is too shallow for the ball because somehow the ball has been able to stay in the socket. Interestingly, the body's adaptation to the lack of a bony containment of the ball is to create whatever else it has at its disposal, which is an enlarged rubbery labrum that, for example, should be half an inch wide, but now has become one inch wide.

Femoroacetabular Impingement (FAI)

Femoro refers to your femur or thigh bone; *acetabular* refers to your hip socket, the acetabulum. *Impingement* means to have an effect upon or to strike, especially with a sharp collision. Thus you can imagine why you have hip pain if this is your diagnosis. Your femur and your acetabulum are banging into each other, and your labrum is probably being damaged between them with every blow.

The Newest Diagnosis

"The eyes don't see what the mind doesn't know" was something Dr. Chit Ranawat taught me during my training at the Hospital for Special Surgery in New York. When Lynda Huey and I wrote our first edition of *Heal Your Hips* in 1999, we didn't know about FAI—in fact, that name didn't exist yet. Since we didn't know about it, we didn't see it on the X-rays or MRIs. We're happy to add this new diagnosis to our list of hip problems. Now that we can see it, we can fix it.

—Robert Klapper, MD

In 2003, the new diagnosis of femoroacetabular impingement (FAI) was identified and given a name by doctors in Switzerland. That proved to be a true game changer in hip preservation. In effect, the identification of FAI created a new subcategory of hip diagnoses, most of which could be solved arthroscopically rather than with a larger open procedure. This was great news for those with hip impingement. In the past decade three types of impingement have been identified, each with a specific arthroscopic solution that trims out small amounts of the offending bone that is causing the impingement and leaves behind a smoothly functioning joint. Without such surgery, the impingement often tears the labrum, which was little understood until recently. The labrum is now considered a crucial part of the hip that must be preserved or reconstructed.

FAI is a major source of hip pain. Since we can now identify it and treat it, the level of sophistication in treating hip problems has risen. Learn the latest, in-depth information about FAI in chapter 5.

Posttraumatic Osteoarthritis

Posttraumatic osteoarthritis is virtually the same thing as osteoarthritis except that it is caused by previous structural damage. The damage doesn't have to be in the hip either. Trauma to an ankle or a knee that leads to a leg-length discrepancy can lead to arthritis of a hip. Injury to any weight-bearing joint—the lower back, the hip, knee, foot, or ankle—can cause eventual damage to adjacent joints. In fact, the injury doesn't even have to be on the same leg. A right knee injury could cause problems with a left hip. If you fractured your leg or even your ankle years ago, that may have altered your gait such that you became arthritic in your hip.

A former professional basketball player had knee surgery that left his knee unable to straighten completely. Several things began to happen over the next few years. The muscles surrounding the knee could no longer go through their full range of motion, so they began to atrophy (decrease in size) even though this athlete worked extensively in the pool and in the weight room. Since the knee couldn't straighten, that leg functioned as if it were shorter and caused him to limp. Next, this athlete began bending at the hip when he walked to accommodate the abnormal function of his knee. Thus he began using his hip joint abnormally too. The hip joint was no longer going through its full range of motion, and the same deterioration process began, first of the muscles, then of the other soft tissues surrounding the hip, and finally of the joint itself. His hip became damaged not because of trauma to the hip but because of trauma to the knee.

This is probably the easiest of all the categories of hip problems to diagnose, unless of course you've forgotten about childhood or adolescent injuries that could be the cause of today's orthopedic problems. Carefully complete the physical history questionnaire in chapter 3, and perhaps you'll find clues regarding your current hip condition.

Let's say you broke your hip as a child or a teenager. Doctors fixed it, but let's use KlapperVision to look at how it was "fixed." Imagine throwing a teacup onto a concrete floor and seeing it smash into pieces. Even if you used the best glue possible and managed to reconstruct the cup perfectly, you would still see dozens of seams. Surgeons may have put your hip back together with plates and screws and whatever else it took to reconstruct the normal anatomy, but even so, your body knows the difference. Years later, the irregularities in your anatomy begin to behave like very fine sandpaper; in the long run, they are enough to wear out the joint.

The symptoms of posttraumatic osteoarthritis are nearly the same as those of osteoarthritis. The only significant difference is that if surgery has taken place, your pain could be coming from the plates and screws that were used to reconstruct the hip or femur or pelvis. The tip of a piece of metal could be sticking into a muscle or other soft tissue, causing inflammation. In that case, removing the hardware could relieve your pain.

Avascular Necrosis (AVN)

The *a-* part of avascular necrosis means without. *Vascular* means blood supply. *Necrosis* means death. So avascular necrosis, or AVN, is death to the bone because of an absent blood supply.

KlapperVision: Think of your hip joint as a lake in the mountains. Some lakes have multiple streams that come down through the mountains to feed them, keeping the lakes full of water. Then consider a lake fed by only one stream. If you were to block one of the streams to a lake that has multiple streams feeding it, there wouldn't be much effect. It would still have what is known as **collateral circulation**: it's getting water from other sources, not just one. But if you were to block the stream to a lake that has only the one water source, the lake would go dry.

The hip joint, unlike other parts of your body, is like the lake that has only one stream feeding it. Drawing 2-7 shows the one major blood vessel into the hip joint. If that vessel is damaged in any way, your hip will lose its nourishing source to the bone, its blood supply, and it will die. Notice how the head of the femur has collapsed due to the death of the bone under the cartilage surface.

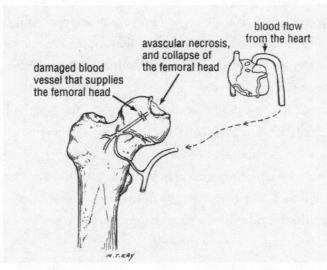

Drawing 2-7. Collapse of head of femur due to loss of blood supply.

Trauma is a common cause of avascular necrosis of the hip. If you were in a sports accident or a car wreck and the femoral head or neck was broken, the blood vessel could have been torn, causing AVN. If you dislocated your hip, the ball went outside the socket and the blood vessels were stretched. The hip has to be put back into place within six to twelve hours. The longer the hip is out of position, the longer the blood vessels to the hip are being stretched, and the greater the chance that the hip will die. With every hip dislocation, you're hoping the blood vessels were stretched, not torn, but you won't know for sure until some time goes by. You may see bone death right away or over time, but nearly always you'll see it within three months if it is going to occur.

Certain drugs can also cause AVN: steroids such as prednisone and cortisone are the main culprits. These drugs are often used for the treatment of asthma, cancer, and skin disorders. Most cases arise from long-term use of these medications, but there have been occasional cases that show no matter how the drug got into your system—by intravenous injection or by mouth—it can cause serious negative side effects, including AVN. In the 1990s, we started seeing AVN patients who were taking protease inhibitor drugs to combat HIV. That family of drugs has been shown to have the side effect of causing AVN in hips.

In pharmacology we refer to drugs as being idiosyncratic in terms of people's responses to them. Two different people can take the same pill and can have similar or opposing reactions to it. One may take the drug with little or no side effects while the other may get stomach cramps and have allergic reactions. *Never take any medicine without your doctor's advice and without considering its possible effects.*

Alcoholism can be another cause of AVN. Drinking excessive alcohol causes blood cells to form large clumps that move slowly through the vessels or even block them. The longer you remain an alcoholic, the greater your chance of developing avascular necrosis. Working for long periods as a scuba diver also has its dangers: if you contract the bends, a condition in which oxygen and nitrogen bubbles form in the bloodstream, you can cause damage to the hip's precious blood supply and develop AVN.

The symptoms of avascular necrosis usually include severe hip pain that comes on abruptly. A sudden absence of blood supply can cause an immediate, acute feeling of intense pain. Interestingly, the pain can be most intense in the beginning and decrease thereafter. Other symptoms include groin pain that goes down the front of your thigh and pain when rotating your leg side to side. *It's important to see your doctor right away.*

Soft-Tissue Injuries

The most common soft-tissue injuries are:

- Tendinitis
- Muscle strains
- Bursitis
- Capsulitis
- Ligament strains
- Muscle and capsule contractures

Tendinitis. Tendinitis is inflammation of the tendon that attaches muscles to bones. It feels like a sharp, sticking pain whenever the muscle is contracted and can occur because of overuse or overstretching of a muscle. It can also be due to trauma: the tendon may be strained or partially torn. Hip-flexor tendons, located up high at the front of the thigh, and the gluteal tendons where the buttocks meet the hamstrings are the two most common locations of tendinitis in the hip area. You can usually find the sore tendon by palpating (probing) the tissues with the fingers.

Muscle strains. Muscle strain is the tearing of muscle fibers. Strains can be mild or severe, depending on how many fibers are torn. The adductors and hamstrings are the most common muscles around the hip to be strained.

Bursitis. Bursitis, generally caused by trauma, impact, or overuse of the hip, is the inflammation of the bursae, or protective sacklike cushions in the joint. You may feel a sharp pain on the outside of your hip whether you are moving your hip or not.

Capsulitis. Capsulitis is an inflammation of the capsule that surrounds the hip joint. It creates a very deep hip pain that you feel whenever you move. Capsulitis can be due to trauma, overuse, or degenerative changes inside the joint.

Ligament strains. Deep in the hip, around the joint, are the ligaments that reinforce the integrity of the structure and keep it solidly together. It takes fairly severe trauma to the hip to damage those deep, ropelike ligaments, trauma of the magnitude of a car accident or a bad fall.

Muscle and capsule contractures. A muscle contracture is a persistent shortening of a muscle; a capsule contracture is the constriction of a joint capsule. The result of either is deep, sharp, restrictive pain and limited movement of the hip. The most common limitation is a hip-flexor contracture in which the hip remains slightly bent at all times; further, the buttocks above the sore hip will lose strength and tone.

Rheumatoid Arthritis (RA)

Rheumatoid arthritis (RA) is an autoimmune disease in which the body's immune system attacks its own tissues. It is passed on genetically. For whatever reason, a miscalculation or perhaps a defect in the **DNA**, the immune system falsely identifies its own tissues as foreign substances and begins to attack them as if they were a bacteria or other invader to be eliminated. KlapperVision: picture the redness and reaction of a bee sting or a splinter.

RA affects more than two million North Americans each year, the majority of whom are women. In fact, RA strikes women three times as often as it does men. In its mildest form, its symptoms include joint discomfort, but if it progresses to its most serious form, it can cause painfully deformed joints and even harm the body's organs. The onset of this disease is typically between the ages of twenty and forty, which means that women are usually affected during their childbearing years.

All joints are lined with a **synovial membrane**, which is a two-layer membrane on a bed of fat, composed of cells that normally produce **synovial fluid**. Synovial fluid is a transparent fluid resembling egg white. It is found in joint cavities, tendon sheaths, and **bursae**. When working normally, this fluid lubricates and feeds cartilage surfaces. In RA, the synovial cells that line the joint leak a corrosive enzyme that acts like battery acid on the tissue it encounters. The enzyme's damage to the cartilage is devastating: in effect, it peels the cartilage away, making it thinner on the periphery of the joint. KlapperVision: Imagine a scoop of ice cream sitting in an ice-cream cone. The scoop of ice cream is the ball and the cone is the socket. The damage from the corrosive enzyme occurs where the cone meets the ice cream. The areas that are damaged are called **periarticular erosions**. (In Greek, *peri* means around, or the perimeter.) These periarticular erosions start on the line around the joint rather than at the dome of the socket because that's where a large number of synovial cells are found. It's the **synovium** that destroys cartilage, so that's where the cartilage damage occurs first. As the erosion continues, it eats its way toward the top of the dome. A classic way of diagnosing RA is to see a reduction in total bone mass, called **osteoporosis**, showing up as washed-out-looking bone on a patient's X-rays along with the defects and crevices where the cartilage stops and the regular bone begins—periarticular erosions.

Osteoporosis can also be caused by the medicine RA patients take. Or by disuse! If the pain of swollen and inflamed joints causes patients to cease their normal activities, or to start limping, they are no longer putting a full load on their bones. That's a signal to the body that there's little stress on the bones, so the body starts to reabsorb more bone from the joints and the surrounding bones.

The bottom line with RA is that the joint lining is destroying the joint. All areas that have lubricating surfaces get involved: that means the tendons, ligaments, and cartilage are all affected. Often you'll see deformity taking place in the hands of RA patients. Where osteoarthritis causes a knobby type of knuckles called Heberden's nodes, RA patients will often get an angulation to their hands so that the fingers point to the outside. Their fingers, wrists, and hands can be irregularly shaped in many different ways. (The French artist Renoir was thought to have RA because the hands that he painted, probably while looking at his own, showed these deformities in the works he painted in his later years.)

Early symptoms of rheumatoid arthritis include joint swelling and pain with no history of trauma or infection. Later, rheumatoid nodules can form at the tips of the elbows and on the feet and knees. These fatty bumps are under the skin and can become debilitating if they cause the skin to break down. If other diagnoses have been ruled out for your hip problem, it may be the systemic disease RA. This can be diagnosed simply by a blood test by a rheumatologist.

In spite of the many things that can go wrong with hips, there are steps you can take to alleviate the pain and limited function that accompany these various conditions. As you reach the right diagnosis in chapter 3, you can immediately begin treatments suggested in chapter 6, then start the pool and land programs in chapters 9 and 12.

3

THE RIGHT DIAGNOSIS

Times have changed. People no longer need to rely solely on their doctors for medical knowledge. Today we live in an information age when anyone can discover, with the click of a computer's mouse, the latest developments in the diagnosis and treatment of medical conditions. And because you are reading this book, you're now one of the many who are making an effort to understand their own hip problems.

Hip Help

To be your hip's best friend, keep up with the latest research on new hip treatments and regularly check the latest information we make available on our website: www.hiphelp.com.

—Robert Klapper, MD

A Written Physical History

A good way to continue delving for information is to prepare a physical history. Use the form that follows to trigger your thinking. Go over each item carefully, and as you do, you'll probably surprise yourself by remembering events of years ago. You may also think of details not included on the form. Write them down. Begin to keep track day by day of your pain: how often your hip hurts, what time of day it seems to hurt most, and what kinds of things you do that relieve the pain.

A caution: People often say that their hip pain "came out of nowhere." Such statements offer no help in a diagnosis. Better to think hard about the recent past, about a fall or other event that could have damaged 95 percent of one of the structures of your hip. No pain ensued at the time, but weeks or even months later, when the other 5 percent of that same portion of the hip was damaged by something as simple as bending to pick a flower, pain began. With such lag time between the inciting event and hip pain, your job becomes that of a detective. Dig back into the past. It's easy to forget a fall from a ladder or a slip off a curb if no pain resulted. Yet most of the injury could have been caused at that earlier time.

A final caution: Don't overlook a remembered pain that was once acute but then vanished and never returned! To understand how this could have happened, consider an analogy: A woman starts a new gardening activity that strenuously uses her hands and develops a blister on her palm that causes acute pain. She gives the blister a few days to heal, then continues gardening off and on over the next months. The blister eventually turns into a callus, the pain completely deadened.

Remembering such a previous flare-up of hip pain can greatly help in diagnosing your condition.

Physical History

What is your hip problem?
___Pain
___Limping, but no pain
___Faulty gait or walking pattern
___Limited movement

What is the location of your pain? (Circle all that apply.)

	L = Left	R = Right	B = Both
Side of the hip	L	R	B
Lower back	L	R	B
Groin	L	R	B
Thigh	L	R	B
Knee	L	R	B
Foot	L	R	B

When did the pain start?

___After trauma

___After a heavy workout

___After a fall

___Gradual in onset with no specific beginning date

___Other, explain _____

_____

Have you had a problem with your hip(s) in the past?

___As a child

___Wore leg braces as a child

___As a teenager

___New problem

___Other, explain _____

_____

Is your hip problem associated with work or the exercises you're doing? _____

_____

What relieves the pain? _____

_____

What makes it worse? _____

_____

*What medications are you currently taking? (Please include aspirin, over-the-counter
medications, birth control pills, supplements, etc.)* _____

_____

_____

_____

Have you taken any new medication(s) in the last year? _____
_____

Have you had prior treatment, tests, or diagnoses on your hip(s)?

___In the past year

___Many years ago

    Please be specific _____

    _____

What have you done for the pain?

___Nothing yet

___Visiting doctor

___Taken anti-inflammatories (aspirin, Motrin, Advil)

___Changed fitness routine

___Ceased exercise program

___Using a cane

___Using crutches

___Using a wheelchair

Do you drink alcohol? Yes ___ No ___

___Occasional social drinker

___Several drinks every evening

___Alcohol intake has gone down in the past year

___Alcohol intake has gone up in the past year

Has your environment changed in the past year?

___Started working

___Stopped working

___Changed jobs

___Moved to a new home

___House has more stairs

___Office has more stairs

Have you moved to a new climate? Yes __ No __

   ___Moved from humid climate to dry

   ___Moved from dry climate to humid

Have you begun wearing new shoes? Explain. _____

_____

Are you exercising on a different type of terrain (grass, dirt, asphalt)? _____

_____

Have you had recent surgery or pain involving other parts of your body? _____

_____

How is the rest of your health? _____

_____

Have you had recent weight changes?

   Loss of _____pounds in the past _____months

   Gain of _____pounds in the past _____months

   ___No change in weight

Has anything changed in your driving habits?

   ___New car

   ___Longer commute

   ___Shorter commute

Has anything changed in your sexual habits?

   ___Pain during sex

   ___Increased activity

   ___Decreased activity

Have you had a recent increase in travel?

___Increased air travel

___Increased car travel

___Increased train travel

Have your sleep patterns recently changed?

___Increased due to lack of energy

___Decreased due to pain

___Erratic due to intermittent pain

Do you scuba dive?

___Never

___Occasionally

___Regularly

___History of any long scuba dives or diving accidents

Have you changed your diet? If so, how? _____

_____

Are you having trouble with the activities of daily living?

___Walking

___Going up and down stairs

___Getting in and out of the car

___Putting on and taking off shoes and socks

___Getting up and down from a sofa or chair

___Other, list _____

_____

The Home Self-Examination

Once you've completed your written history, sit facing a full-length mirror for a self-examination. Breathe comfortably and relax until you feel you are sitting as you normally would.

Notice whether both your feet are pointing straight forward or whether one or both of your feet are externally rotated (turned outward) further than usual. Look for a "Charlie Chaplin" foot placement, the opposite of pigeon-toed. If your right foot, for instance, is pointing toward the right rather than straight ahead, we would say your right leg is externally rotated. Perhaps both of your feet have pointed outward ever since you can remember. In this case, noticing external rotation may not be significant. But if you've never been aware of external rotation and now you see just one foot pointing outward, this becomes significant: it may be an early sign of arthritis in your hip. Even if you have no pain in your hip to indicate the beginning of a problem, this may be a silent signal that your hip no longer has its normal rotational capability and that the surrounding soft tissues are becoming affected.

Inspect the way your shoes are wearing. Your shoes are like the tires on your car; they can tell you if your alignment is off. So notice if there's a difference between one shoe and the other. Notice if you're wearing through your newest shoes faster and in a pattern different from your usual wear pattern. This subtle difference could be an early indicator of arthritic changes in your hip joint or problems with the soft tissues surrounding the joint.

Watch yourself in the mirror as you take off your shoes and socks. See if you're making abnormal movements. Is it difficult or impossible for you to bend your hips enough to reach your foot? Does your knee have to turn outward so you can remove your shoe? Are you "cheating" by using your other foot rather than bending down to remove your shoes or socks? If you find abnormalities in these movements, they could indicate restrictions of movement in your hip.

Assess your toenails. Do they look in need of care because you aren't able to bend enough at the hip to maintain hygiene and keep them clipped? This is another silent symptom of hip problems.

Wearing only your bathing suit or underwear, stand and look at yourself in a full-length mirror. Are you standing straight or are you leaning? Do you have most of your weight on one leg? A hip contracture (a soft-tissue condition) may have you standing most comfortably on one leg with the other one slightly bent. A leg-length discrepancy could have you leaning to one side.

Get dressed and go up and down some nearby stairs. Are you able to **reciprocate** the stairs; that is, are you able to put your right foot on one step, your left foot on the next step, and continue in that manner? Or are you putting your right foot on a step, and then putting your left foot on the same step in order to advance? A healthy hip is able to reciprocate going both upstairs and downstairs. Losing the ability to reciprocate stairs is one of the first changes in your gait you'll notice if your hip is unhealthy.

The Home Exam with a Friend or Family Member

You may be walking abnormally, but because you've been doing so for weeks or even months, you no longer notice. You may also have become accustomed to having slightly swollen ankles or knees, so ask someone whose judgment you trust to help with this portion of the exam; wear shorts to allow your partner to examine your knees and ankles.

Wearing athletic shoes, walk back and forth so that your friend can observe you from the front, the back, and the side. Your friend will be able to tell if you are limping. If you are lurching or swaying from side to side, you have what's called an **antalgic gait**—an abnormal walking pattern that is due to pain. More specifically, it's a **coxalgic gait**, meaning the abnormal gait is due to hip pain. When you put weight on the hip that hurts, your body automatically compensates and makes an effort to take the weight quickly off that leg. If your friend is seeing this coxalgic gait, but you have no hip pain, the abnormal movement is probably being caused by weak abductor muscles on the outside of your hip.

If your friend sees your head bobbing up and down as you walk, that probably means you have what is called a **short-leg gait**. One of your legs might be longer or shorter in length because of arthritis, because of a fracture, or because one leg was shorter at birth. If the the femur (thigh bone) was badly fractured, the leg may have shortened when the two ends of the bone were brought together to heal. In some hip dysplasia cases, the ball is no longer in the socket. Instead, it's functioning somewhere near the socket, above or below, and that, of course, changes the length of the leg.

One of your legs could be shorter because a scoliosis (curvature of the spine) is forcing your pelvis to rotate, creating a leg that functions as though it were short even if it isn't anatomically shorter. Nearly all humans have a slight leg-length discrepancy, but a half-inch difference or more is usually necessary before a short-leg gait can be seen.

Remove your shoes and socks. Ask your friend to check for any swelling in either of your ankles or knees. Since you can't see swelling in the hip because big muscles surround that area, you look instead for swelling of the nearby joints. If both knees and both ankles are swollen, that could be caused by a problem with your heart. If only one of the four joints inspected is swollen, that often indicates a problem within that specific joint or a blockage of the blood flow to that leg. If one entire leg seems swollen, that could reflect problems in that hip. The irony is that you won't see the swelling in the hip, the actual site of damage; you'll see it "downstream," in the joints and tissue below.

Seeking Help from a Doctor

Once you've completed the written history and the self-exam and taken time to consider your answers, you're prepared to help your doctor diagnose and treat your affected hip; that is, if you've decided to consult a doctor. Your reason for doing so may be as hard to describe as your "sixth sense." Or your reason may depend entirely on the strength and duration of your pain, the loss of sleep due to pain, the restriction of your daily activities because of the soreness of your hip joint, or the alteration of your gait—at some point along the continuum of hip symptoms, you'll decide to seek relief by combining your knowledge with a doctor's.

You May Need to Insist on an MRI

In years past, an X-ray was enough to get complete information about your hip problem, but not any longer. Your **HMO** may not be eager to offer you an expensive MRI (see chapter 4). And yet the new diagnosis of FAI is often seen only on an MRI. You will want to persuade your doctor and your insurance company that you need one, because if you wait to see FAI on an X-ray, it may be too late—you may have missed the window where a minor arthroscopic procedure could help you. The most complicated cases may need an MR Arthrogram (MRA) to spot FAI or a potential labral tear.

If we catch these problems early enough, we can work to resolve a torn labrum in the pool without surgery or, if needed, remove the bony impingement and reconstruct the labrum arthroscopically. You want to know if you have FAI, so **don't let your primary care doctor or the insurance company deny you an MRI.** This doesn't mean every patient needs an MRI. But if you've been working for several months to reduce your hip pain and regain your strength and flexibility and it hasn't changed significantly, don't let your doctor tell you that you're fine just because your X-ray looks normal. Our goal is to empower you with the knowledge of what needs to be done. Your doctor may not yet understand this new, sophisticated diagnosis of FAI. Read chapter 4 about X-rays, MRIs, and MRAs and chapter 5 on FAI. The more you know, the more you can confidently be your own advocate.

—Robert Klapper, MD

Schedule an office visit with your doctor. He or she will have you get an X-ray, MRI, or both. Take along your written history for discussion during your initial office visit. For the moment, let me be your doctor. In the following items, I've summarized the possible implications of your history.

Symptoms

How long have you had hip problems? Weeks? Months? Did the problem start suddenly or come on gradually? Is the pain associated with an acute event, an accident or injury, or has the problem been slowly progressing? The location of the pain and the length of time it has existed will help in making a correct diagnosis.

Exacerbating Factors

When you've been sitting in a chair or lying in bed, do you feel a sharp pain in the groin or hip area when you stand and take your first steps? This is called **starting pain** and is considered **pathognomonic** to hip problems. Pathognomonic symptoms are the equivalent of a bull's-eye, the real signal that indeed you have a problem in your hip and not elsewhere.

Picture an auto mechanic in a small-town gas station. As you drive your car in, it's making a noise, and from across the garage the mechanic says, "It's your intake manifold, and spark plug number four needs to be changed." He hears in the way the car is idling what's wrong. The sound is pathognomonic to him. That's what starting pain is to hip problems.

Does your favorite workout or sport make your hip sore? Does the pain go away when you cut back on your recreational activities? You may have to choose your sports and workouts with more consideration for your hip. Chapter 7 will show you how to limit abusive activities you enjoy and help you cross-train with nurturing ones that won't aggravate your hip.

Do you have hip pain after walking a certain length of time? When you sit down, does the pain go away? Answers to these questions can tell whether this is a circulatory or neurological problem. If your hip pain worsens as you walk but goes away completely when you sit down, that may indicate a circulatory problem. If, however, the pain in your hip and legs gets worse as you walk and does not go away when you sit to rest, that might indicate a neurological condition such as a herniated disk or a pinched nerve.

Medications

Discuss with your doctor the medications and supplements you are currently taking: prescription drugs, aspirin and other over-the-counter pain relievers, hormone replacement, wellness supplements, amino acids, calcium, vitamin C, multivitamins, and birth control pills. Are you having side effects? Do you know which medicine or supplement is causing which effect? Have you taken any prednisone, oral cortisone, or other corticosteroids that may have caused your hip problem? Your dermatologist may have given you steroids for an outbreak of poison oak. Your eye doctor may have given you oral steroids for chronic conjunctivitis or other eye conditions. All this information is vital.

Deep joint destruction that erodes the cartilage and leaves the bone exposed can cause nerve pain. This kind of pain can't be relieved except by narcotics (codeine, for example), which mask all pain. If taking an over-the-counter anti-inflammatory can reduce some of the pain in your hip joint, that's a good sign that such severe destruction hasn't yet occurred; thus you might be a candidate for conservative treatment.

Prior Treatment

Have you seen another doctor or therapist for this hip condition? Have you had previous therapy, tests, or diagnoses? Have you had previous hip surgery or fractures? Did you have hip problems in childhood?

If you had surgery in childhood and an infection developed in any of the bones near your hip, that would be important to know, even if the infection was treated successfully. That infection may have destroyed some of the bone or the growth plate at the end of the bone—destruction that can lead to problems later on. If you have a poor recollection of your childhood, talk to your parents, siblings, or other relatives. If any of them have memories of your having had surgery or wearing a brace as a child, you owe it to yourself to get an X-ray. Then you will know the status of your hip.

In the more recent past, you may have seen various doctors or therapists for your ongoing hip problem. The solution to one problem in your body in the past may now be the cause of your current hip problem. You need to assemble all the previous information you have gathered about your hip to give to your current doctor so you won't have to start the process all over again. Do your best to understand the conclusions other doctors have reached in order to summarize them during your conversation with your new doctor.

Sleep Pattern

Does hip pain keep you awake at night?

Because 40 percent of your body weight goes through the hip joint as you roll around in bed, a sore hip will wake people more often than any other joint. Such sleep deprivation is usually the end stage of the progression of hip problems: once hip pain starts affecting sleep, people who were reluctant to contact a doctor will now do so.

> ### *Attention Weekend Warriors: Be a Reader-Warrior!*
>
> We've got reader-warriors out there who have read our book and they are empowered like nobody else to ask the right questions.
>
> —Robert Klapper, MD

Functional Assessment

How well are you functioning in your daily life in spite of the problems you're having with your hip? Can you walk up and down stairs? Can you get in and out of a car? Do you need a cane to move smoothly throughout the day?

I watch my patients move around the office so I can have a glimpse of what their daily hip-life is like. I watch how quickly or slowly they move, how they take their shoes off, how they get up from the chair. Do they grimace in pain as they stand up? I watch these things not because patients might be hiding something from me, but because I can sometimes see more in their movements than they can see themselves. They've made lifestyle changes, adaptations of movement that they no longer notice.

The Doctor's Physical Exam

Following this conference on your written history, ask your doctor to examine your entire body. Here is the way I examine my patients, beginning with gait.

Gait

I ask patients to walk down the hall so I can see how fast they move. I watch to see if they're limiting or shortening their steps or if they're leaning to one side. I notice if one foot is turned out or if both are. If the patient is limping, it's for one or more of these reasons: leg-length discrepancy, pain, or weakness of the abductor muscles.

Leg Length

Have you ever had a fracture of any of the bones of the leg or hip? Does one hemline of your pants appear longer than the other?

To measure leg length, I face the patient, who is standing barefoot in front of me. I place my hands on the top of his iliac crests (the top of the pelvis), as shown in Photo 3-1. My hands should be at the same level. If one is higher than the other, I have the patient step on blocks or lifts of differing heights until his hips are at the same height. If, when he stands on a quarter-inch block, his hips are level, he has a quarter-inch leg-length discrepancy. If there's more than a half-inch difference between the length of the two legs, I ask the patient to wear a lift in the shoe of the shorter leg in order to create better balance. If the discrepancy is less than half an inch, I tell the patient not to use lifts. If they aren't really needed, lifts can create back problems and hip problems. In my opinion, your body is better off without shoe lifts to cope with slight differences.

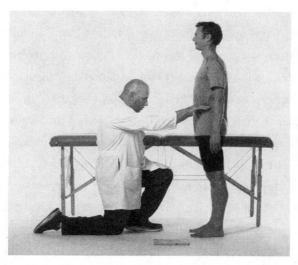

Photo 3-1. Measuring a leg-length discrepancy.

Is Hip Pain Coming from Your Spine?

Many patients come to see me who have both an arthritic spine and an arthritic hip. This is a difficult diagnostic dilemma—is your back causing hip pain or is it your hip causing the hip pain even though you have an arthritic back? Unfortunately, I have seen many people who have had spine surgery and their hip pain persists. This is an important pot hole to avoid.

A simple, elegant test called a lidocaine test places an injection of numbing medicine into the hip under X-ray guidance to make sure it has accurately gone into the joint. For the next three hours, you should do movements that you know would ordinarily hurt your hip: go up and down some stairs, dance, get in and out of your car, or whatever else you know would cause pain. During those three hours when the lidocaine is working to numb all of your hip pain, you should be pain free. If you are, numbing your hip with the lidocaine test proves that your hip is the source of your pain. But if you have the same pain despite numbing your hip, you wouldn't have hip surgery. Your spine is the source of your pain.

Examination of the Knees

It's extremely unusual for patients who have bad knees to be feeling pain in their hips. What often happens, however, is that patients tell me they have knee problems when, in fact, the problem is really coming from their hips. They feel pain down the front of the thigh that's emanating from the hip. Here's my theory on why this happens: The big muscles that run down the front of the thigh and into the kneecap are called the **quadriceps** muscles. *Quad* means four in Latin, and there are four muscles in the quadriceps group. One of the most powerful members of the quadriceps group is the rectus femoris. It is the most "superficial," meaning it is the closest to the surface. Drawing 3-1 shows that it has two heads, or two attachment sites. The first head is attached to the pelvis, but there's a deeper anchoring site for the second head, or the reflected head. It attaches close to the front of the hip joint capsule. If there's some heat or pain in the joint, it can sometimes radiate down the whole rectus femoris muscle because one of the muscle's origin sites is sitting on an inflamed area. This means that patients who have an inflamed hip joint capsule often feel deep pain down the fronts of their thighs and are misled into thinking they have a knee problem instead of a hip problem. So don't be fooled by knee pain.

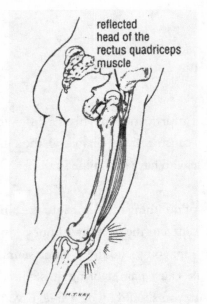

reflected head of the rectus quadriceps muscle

Drawing 3-1. The reflected head of the rectus femoris can cause knee pain.

As the patient lies on the exam table, I examine one knee and then the other. I assess the ligament integrity, range of motion, and the tracking mechanism—how well the kneecap rides within the groove of the femur. I check for a grinding sensation called **crepitus**. If the patient feels pain in either knee, we try to find its specific location. The most important thing is to discover if the pain is along the joint line of the knee. I ask the patient to bend his knees to a 90-degree angle; then I feel the kneecap. I feel the outline of it; then I feel the bottom portion of the kneecap, which roughly corresponds to the joint line. I slide my index and middle fingers across the joint line to the outside and to the inside. If there's tenderness in that area, this patient may have a problem with the shock-absorbing cartilage (**meniscus**) inside the knee joint. The meniscus could be torn or there could be early arthritic changes starting inside the knee joint. Pain, swelling, and limited movement in knees can also be caused by compensating for poor gait mechanics that come from a sore hip.

Range of Motion of the Hips

The hip is capable of flexion, extension, rotation, abduction, and adduction. (See Drawings 2-3 to 2-6 on page 20.) During our examination we assess all these planes of motion in order to determine whether there are any restrictions.

Flexion and extension. To evaluate the flexion of a patient's hip, I ask him to pull both knees to his chest. Normally one knee will be pulled closer to the chest than the other because the sore hip can't bend as well. I ask the patient to pull the knee on the healthier leg as close to the chest as possible and look at the amount of flexion that's possible. Then we compare that to the painful side. To check extension, I have the patient continue holding one leg while lowering the other leg straight onto the table. If the leg doesn't go all the way down, (see Photo 3-2) the patient has a hip flexor contracture, which means that his hip is being held in a slightly flexed position by the soft tissues surrounding the hip. Either the muscles or the joint capsule are constricted and won't allow the hip to extend fully onto the table.

Here's how this constriction happens: When your hip joint doesn't move well through its entire range of motion, the muscles around it are no longer being stretched to their full movement. The affected muscles become fixed in their shortened state and are called muscle contractures.

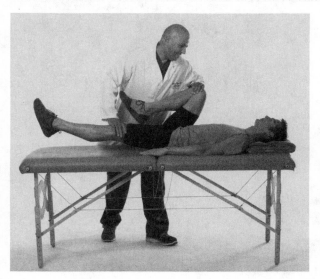

Photo 3-2. Hip flexor contracture.

Rotation. First we look at the healthier hip's internal and external rotation to establish the norm. Then we repeat the measurements on the painful hip. (See these tests being performed in Photos 3-4 and 3-5 on page 52.) I test for external rotation by bending the patient's knee and seeing how far I can move his knee as if he were going to sit cross-legged in a yoga class. If his knee is facing straight up and I can't turn it at all to the side, that's 0 degrees. If his knee can turn so far that his thigh is parallel with the table, that's 90 degrees. The average person has between 40 and 70 degrees of external rotation.

Next we turn the leg in the other direction. The knee turns in and the foot angles outward, forcing the hip into internal rotation. The norm is different for each of us, but we want to see some internal rotation. We expect to see at least 10 to 20 degrees; 30 degrees would be a lot. This is a significant test because internal rotation is usually the first movement to elicit pain in patients with an arthritic hip.

Test for FAI and a torn labrum. The exam for impingement (FAI) and a torn labrum is flexion plus internal rotation. I flex the patient's knee and hip to a maximum amount of flexion as in Photo 3-3 and ask if there's any pain in the groin. I then externally rotate the hip so that the foot crosses the other leg and the knee is out to the side as in Photo 3-4. I ask if there's any pain in the groin. Usually patients say no to both of these. Now I flex the knee and turn the knee in the opposite direction. The knee turns across the body into internal rotation as in Photo 3-5. If flexion and maximal internal rotation elicits pain in the groin, the patient usually has a torn labrum.

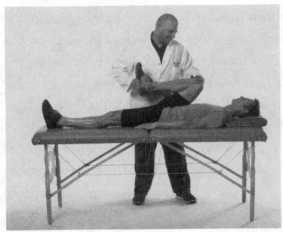

Photo 3-3. Knee and hip are in maximal flexion.

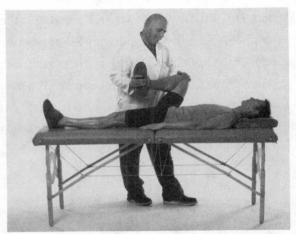

Photo 3-4. Hip with flexion and external rotation.

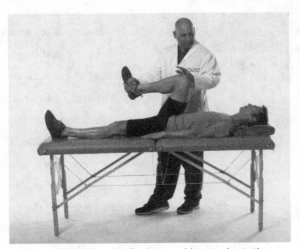

Photo 3-5. Hip with flexion and internal rotation.

That is the classic exam for impingement where either the neck of the femur or the edge of the socket is pinching the labrum. (Review page 25 for more information about labral tears and see chapter 5 for a thorough explanation of FAI.) Since the labrum is rich in pain fibers, groin pain in this position means the exam is positive for a torn labrum. We can't tell which side of the socket is causing the impingement that has torn the labrum until we get more information from an MRI or MR arthrogram (MRA). See chapter 4 for explanations of these tests.

Abduction and adduction. When you **abduct** your leg, you move it away from the body and directly to the side. To test for abduction, I pull the patient's leg wide to the side.

When you **adduct** your leg, you are bringing your leg back to or across the midline of your body. I put my hand on one of the bony prominences of the pelvis to feel whether the whole pelvis is rocking with the movement. I want to feel for myself whether the patient is getting movement because the hip is functioning or because the lower back and pelvis are moving. I want to see if there's any lack of hip-joint function.

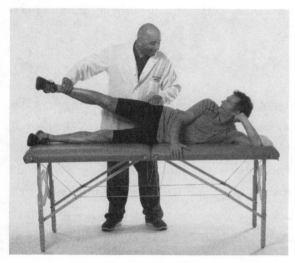

Photo 3-6. Test for bursitis.

Bursitis

The patient lies on his side on the exam table with the sore hip pointing toward the ceiling. We make sure the hips and knees are straight. Then I ask the patient to lift his whole leg as shown in Photo 3-6. He resists while I push down on the leg. If he has a single, sharp, discrete pain on the side of his hip while he's trying to resist me, we may have found a hip bursitis.

Ankles

I look at the ankles to assess them for swelling. Swelling could mean that a problem in the hip is disrupting the normal blood flow to and from the ankle. My other major concern is that the swelling might be indicative of a systemic problem such as lupus, rheumatoid arthritis, or a heart problem.

Neurological Exam

The human body has two kinds of nerves: sensory and motor. The sensory nerves transmit sensations from the body to the brain so you know what your body is feeling. The motor nerves transmit your intention to move from the brain to the muscles, causing movement. I test both sets of nerves.

First I test the two sets of sensory nerves, one for light touch and one for deep touch. I brush a piece of paper on the patient's foot to see if he feels it. If he doesn't, I could be picking up an early indication of diabetes. For deep touch, I apply pressure with my fingers on the top of the foot and ask the patient if he can feel it. Then I repeat the procedure on the bottom of the foot. I also check to see if the patient has sensation in the tips of his toes.

After I've checked the sensory nerves, I test the motor nerves. I ask the patient to pull his foot upward and resist me as I try to push the foot down. Then I ask him to do the opposite movement, as though he were pushing down on a gas pedal. Again, I provide resistance and lift up against the patient's force. If one leg is working well and the other isn't, we can probably assume nerve problems rather than muscular weakness.

Pulses

There are two areas in the foot and ankle that represent the overall circulation to the big vessels of the lower extremities. We grade these pulses either Grade 0, Grade 1+, or Grade 2+. The dorsalis pedis pulse is on the top of the foot. The posterior tibial pulse is behind the inner ankle bone called the medial malleolus. If your pulse is absent, you're probably not a candidate for surgery, and you'll need to focus on rehabilitation through exercise. If you and your doctor feel you need surgery to correct your hip anatomy, a vascular surgeon could do noninvasive vascular studies to evaluate the integrity of the blood vessels. Without viable circulation, you would be at tremendous risk for surgery.

The Best Information

It's always appropriate to get a second opinion about your condition. Each health-care provider has a bias toward certain procedures, and you'll want to hear several points of view in order to make the best possible choice for the care of your hip.

4

X-RAYS, CT SCANS, AND MRIS

with Douglas Brown, MD

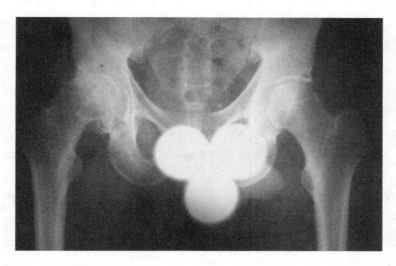

Figure 4-1. A pelvic X-ray. This X-ray is as though a friend is facing you. On your right is a normal hip. Notice the smoothly curving surface on both the ball side and the socket side of the joint. The space between those two surfaces is cartilage. On the left is a hip with osteoarthritis. Notice the rough surfaces and that the cartilage is virtually gone—the two sides look closer together. That means there's no longer a cushion for this joint. The three-lobed white structure in the center is a leaded shield to protect the reproductive organs.

Objective diagnostic tests such as X-rays are the universal language of medicine. I could be in China and unable to converse with another doctor, but as soon as we put up the X-rays, we would both be able to see what was happening in a hip joint. Similarly, once you learn the basics of looking at your X-ray, CT scan, or MRI, you will begin to understand knowledge that is shared universally. In this chapter, I hope to give you the means to explain your hip complaints more clearly to your doctor and better understand his or her diagnosis.

Figure 4-1 shows a pelvic X-ray. The patient's left hip (on the right) is normal, while his right hip (on the left) is not. First, let's look at the normal side. You can see the ball-and-socket joint and the space between the two sides of the joint. Notice the whiteness (the density) of the bone. You'll return to this X-ray several times as you read this chapter.

In the classic teachings of medical school, there are *subjective* complaints of the patient, such as pain, and there are *objective* findings, such as this X-ray. The subjective complaints are things you tell your doctor about where you hurt, how badly you hurt, and how frequently. Although this information is crucial to helping your doctor reach a diagnosis, it is not tangible. But an X-ray is an objective finding you can actually see. So is a CT scan and an MRI. All these tests provide different kinds of information.

A **radiologist** is a medical doctor who has been certified as a specialist in interpreting X-rays and other studies. There are general radiologists and there are sub-specialties within radiology that require advanced training regarding a specific field. In dealing with your hip, the musculoskeletal radiologist will be the most helpful. These are the doctors who will be up-to-date with all the latest findings that are seen on your studies. In 2007, the *American Journal of Radiology* published material that many radiologists had missed in their training—how to identify the new diagnosis of FAI on X-rays, MRIs, and MR arthrograms.

It takes years of training and experience to be able to read an X-ray, CT scan, MRI, or MR arthrogram, so our goal isn't to make you a radiologist, only to demystify a complicated aspect of medicine. This knowledge can have a powerful effect on your body. For instance, scientific experiments routinely use **placebos** to test the effectiveness of drugs. The placebo is merely a sugar or salt pill, but if the person taking it believes it will cure him, many times he gets well. Just as placebos can improve a person's health simply through a belief that the pill is helping, real knowledge can help you visualize your hip problem, understand your options for treatment, and assume responsibility for healing.

Our job is to educate *you* because you may actually be asking questions about a topic that is so new that your own doctor may be unfamiliar with it. If neither your doctor nor your radiologist is familiar with FAI, they won't be talking with you about it as they discuss your diagnosis, because it's not part of their world. If you end up getting an MRI, look in the report. It should say something specific about FAI, even if it's as simple as "No FAI." If not, that's a tip-off that you might need to seek a second opinion and have your studies re-evaluated for this new diagnosis.

These days, state-of-the-art imaging centers use a digital PACS, which stands for Picture Archiving and Communications System. Think of how a digital camera stores pictures on a memory card, yet you can print them onto photo paper if you wish. The PACS works in the same way: digital information from a filmless radiology system is stored at a digital archive, yet can be printed onto plain film or given to you or your doctor electronically. The PACS takes the images, and then, instead of spitting out an X-ray or MRI sheet of film, transmits the data to a workstation in the imaging center for immediate viewing by the radiologist. You'll no longer need to carry a packet of films that can so easily be lost or damaged.

New Technology: Studies Are Never Lost

Until recently, when you had your X-rays taken, that original film was the only information that linked you to your exam. If it was lost or destroyed, it was as if that study was never done because those films could not be brought back—your history was gone. Today, if you lose your images, we can give you a new copy because your information is not stored exclusively where your study was taken—it is also stored in backup locations (digital archives) around the country in case a fire or other catastrophe strikes an imaging center.

PACS systems are available all over the world, but in far greater numbers in the United States and Western Europe. Most major American universities use various PACS systems, all of which are compatible with one another.

—Radiologist Douglas H. Brown, MD

Radiologists can manipulate digital images in several key ways to see more clearly into your hip as they look for the cause of your pain: they can enlarge the image, and they can alter the contrast and the brightness. The resolution on the PACS workstation is excellent, allowing radiologists to enlarge the image to double or triple its original size without losing clarity. Let's say we want to measure the thickness of a hip's cartilage. It will be easier to take that measurement on an enlarged image than on a smaller image. If your study was done on plain film, once that film is printed from an old-style X-ray machine, that's all you've got to work with. Digitally acquired images, however, give the people reading those images much more power in manipulating them for accurate measurements and interpretations.

Another way to manipulate a PACS image is to change its window (contrast) and level (brightness), just as you would on a TV or a computer monitor. When a doctor gets printed film, its window and level are designated by the machine or the technologist at that time. If the films are too light or too dark, there's nothing the doctor can do about it, and he consequently may not be able to see the subtle damage in the hip. But if the films are done on PACS, the window and level can be altered on the workstation to make the contrast sharper and the images darker or lighter, based on the preferences of the person reading the study.

Your orthopedic surgeon will probably have his own X-ray machine, but if an MRI or CT scan is required, you'll most likely be sent elsewhere for those images. Even if your doctor refers you to his favorite imaging center, call to make sure they have a PACS system with the ability to give you an electronic copy or print film as per your doctor's preference. If they don't, find a PACS nearby. If you live in a small town or rural area, it will be worth your travel time to the nearest university to obtain a modern study that lets you store your lifelong health history in a form that is more secure and more adjustable for present and future interpretation. The most advanced technology offers you the best possibility of finding the cause of your pain because once you have an electronic PACS study, you can show it to another doctor or radiologist for a second opinion. The new doctor can manipulate images to his or her own preferences for careful inspection.

No matter where your studies are taken, it's important for you to look at your X-rays and MRIs with your doctor, not to settle for the radiologist's report. This is the time for you to learn about your own hip.

If you might be pregnant, you should not have an X-ray, CT scan, or MRI. Before you have any of these tests, you'll be asked a series of questions to ensure your safety.

Review Your X-Rays with Your Doctor

I enjoy looking at X-rays with my patients and seeing a lightbulb turn on in a patient's mind as the learning process unfolds. I get lucky when only one hip is having problems because then I can say, "Here's a normal hip. This is why. And here's your hip that's bothering you. This is why it's abnormal." But if both hips are bad, I have an example of a normal hip in each of my exam rooms so I can show a patient what normal looks like. Figure 4-1 on page 57 is a classic example.

—Robert Klapper, MD

X-Rays

X-rays use electromagnetic radiation to penetrate solids and create gray-scale images. These images give doctors a look at parts of the body that have density, such as calcium. Bones have calcium, so we see them on X-rays, which are an indispensable tool in the orthopedic examination of a patient, exposing a fracture, dislocation, tumor, or other pathologic changes. Other parts of the body do not contain calcium: cartilage, ligaments, tendons, synovium, labrum, or bursa. Those appear as an empty space on an X-ray. For us to inspect those soft tissues, we use the MRI.

Indicators for Osteoarthritis

We look for these four indicators on an X-ray to diagnose OA:

- Joint space narrowing
- Spurs
- Sclerosis
- Subchondral cysts

Let's suppose you have a normal hip and a problematic hip. When you look at the X-ray of the normal hip, you'll see a space between the ball and the socket of the hip joint. (See Figure 4-1 on page 57.) The space between them isn't air; it's the cartilage at the ends of the bones, but because cartilage doesn't have calcium, it doesn't show up on the X-ray. When you see that wide space on an X-ray, you can conclude there's a healthy cartilage between the ball and the socket. The joint is normal. When you look at the abnormal hip and see the ball getting closer to the socket, that **joint space narrowing** means a loss of cartilage—a loss of joint space, which means arthritis.

You also might see **spurs** (**osteophytes**)—calcified outcroppings on either side of the joint. My opinion is that these spurs are the body's attempt to stabilize the joint when it becomes wobbly from cartilage loss. But spurs actually turn into part of the problem because they are rough growths within the joint where there should be only smooth surfaces. Sometimes pieces of these spurs will break off and become loose bodies, or loose fragments inside the joint.

"Can You Just Get Rid of My Spurs?"

Patients ask me this when we see spurs on their X-rays. So I explain how those spurs probably got there in the first place. As your hip developed in your early years, your ligaments grew to a specific length to cross that joint and tightly stabilize your hip. As arthritis caused the deterioration of the cartilage, the thickness may have decreased by, let's say, half. But your ligaments didn't shrink to maintain their tautness. So the stabilizers can't do their job, and the joint can feel unstable. The ligaments aren't torn; they just aren't functional anymore. So now the bones can rattle around with abnormal movement to the front, back, and side. With each rattle, there is micro-trauma to the ligaments and capsule. Eventually the bone becomes traumatized and bone spurs start to grow. When you understand what spurs represent, you'll see why just removing the spurs is unlikely to lead to a real solution.

—Robert Klapper, MD

Sclerosis is a hardening of the bone. It's the opposite of osteoporosis (fragile bones). Osteoporosis shows up on an X-ray as blacker bone, while sclerosis shows up as denser, whiter-looking bone. As a joint becomes arthritic and begins to have problems functioning smoothly, it no longer shares the weight of the body equally on all its surfaces. You could be limping. The weight bearing becomes concentrated in certain spots of the joint, and those areas become denser: the X-ray will show more sclerosis. Particularly, you'll see sclerosis in avascular necrosis. Without a healthy blood supply, the bone collapses like a sponge and becomes dense as it squashes down.

Subchondral cysts are the fourth indicator of OA. When the cartilage cracks, the synovial joint fluid escapes into the cells in the bone beneath the cartilage and can form pockets of liquid that start to damage the bone and become cysts that can be seen on your X-ray.

Early OA may not be visible on an X-ray, but advanced OA clearly is and would likely show three or four of these indicators. If your X-ray shows these signs of advanced osteoarthritis, your diagnosis will probably be confirmed, and it's unlikely you will need further studies such as a CT scan or MRI.

The X-ray is the best place to start when searching for a diagnosis. It will help your doctor find out if you might have metabolic arthritis (gout), inflammatory arthritis (RA), or degenerative arthritis (OA). An X-ray can also show large things such as AVN or defects that might be associated with FAI, such as a prominent deformity of the femoral head and neck junction. (See Figure 5-1 on page 74.) However, an MRI would be required to see more subtle things to tell if FAI is the underlying source of your hip pain. In effect, an X-ray is the screening study that tells us if you may be a candidate for an MRI.

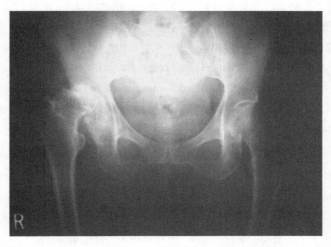

Figure 4-2. X-ray of avascular necrosis. Look at the hip on the left. Notice not only the narrowing of the joint space but also flattening of the spherical head. KlapperVision: the linoleum of your kitchen floor has collapsed because termites have eaten the floorboards below.

MRIs

Magnetic resonance imaging (MRI) does not use X-rays, but rather magnetism and radio waves. The powerful magnet requires certain precautions. If you have a pacemaker, you shouldn't have an MRI because the magnet could interfere with the pacemaker's function. If you've had brain surgery, you'll need to show documentation that metal clips weren't placed inside your brain. If you have tattooed eyeliner, the metal in the tattoo will cause the magnet to tug on your eyelids. This may be mildly painful, so you might want to put an ice pack on your eyes afterward. Other metals in your body, such as rods around the spine or a hip implant, tend not to be magnetic and therefore won't cause problems. You may feel local warming in those areas, but nothing of significance. You'll be asked to remove your keys, watch, hairpins, bra, and jewelry (rings excepted). If you opt to leave your earrings in place, you might feel a mild annoyance as they are pulled on by the magnet.

Make sure you don't have credit cards in your pocket because the magnetic strips will be wiped clean.

The MRI image appears in great detail, using different shades of black, white, and gray to bring out actual tissue types including fat, cartilage, meniscus, tendons, and ligaments. Unlike X-rays and CT scans, the MRI allows us to see both the bones and the soft tissues of the body. This means you can see labral tears, swelling, and inflammation. You won't see any of those things on an X-ray, but they appear readily on an MRI. Bursitis will show up in the area of the bursa as fluid just below the skin. If a herniated disk is the source of your hip pain, you'll be able to see the bulging disk pressing on the nerve that is responsible for sensation and movement in the hip joint.

KlapperVision: To understand the difference between an X-ray and an MRI, imagine that I have a ten-inch-long candle standing upright in a candleholder and that the wick is filled with calcium. If I take an X-ray of that candle, the wax will disappear and the only thing that will show up is the wick running vertically. Now, if I decide I need an MRI of that candle, the image I get of the wick won't be lengthwise, but will instead be a slice right through the candle, and I'll be viewing the wick as if from above. I'll see it sitting like a doughnut hole with the wax as the doughnut all around it. Now I can see the front, back, right, and left sides of the wick, not just the vertical length of it. Further, I can see the individual strands that are braided together diagonally to make up the wick, and I can also see any defects in the wax. There will be a series of "slices" showing up in the pictures so we can search for the problem. We will be able to see, for instance, that there's a disruption of the fibers that make up the wick, or that the fibers have been stretched and are no longer oriented correctly.

Then, to identify the location, I look at a localizer reference grid, which will tell me that the first photograph corresponds to the four-inch height level of the candle and the second photograph corresponds to the eight-inch height level. The MRI can take as many slices as are necessary. The radiologist can request ten slices in a ten-inch candle, or he can request thirty. If, for instance, the radiologist is worried that there might be a tumor in the wick, he can specify thinner cuts, which will provide more pictures and more information.

An X-ray tells us what the wick looks like from only one side, top to bottom, but the MRI gives us a three-dimensional look from above at the entire circumference of the wick and the candle—front, back, left, and right—in the multiple places where it has been sliced.

Treat the Symptoms, Not the Findings

The findings on the MRI should match the symptoms you have. Even if your MRI results say that you've torn your labrum, if your symptoms are subsiding, don't rush into surgery. Doctors can operate when the symptoms require it, but not before. Don't let them operate strictly on the findings of a test!

—Robert Klapper, MD

Sometimes an MRI offers too much information. For instance, if I have to develop a surgical plan to reconstruct a patient's hip, I want the clear, crisp lines of an X-ray to help me understand the geometry and the architecture, not the nebulous lines with all the information an MRI gives me. The X-ray lets me focus on the structure without anything else clouding my vision.

To have an MRI of your hip, you'll go into a room and see a large doughnut-shaped machine. The doughnut hole is a narrow tube more than six feet long. You'll lie flat on your back on a padded, moveable platform that's about as wide as a stretcher with your feet pointed toward the tube. Your feet will be taped together to keep your hips in the correct anatomical position. Your entire body, including your head, will slide inside the tube. The smaller you are, the more comfortable you'll be. A woman five feet five inches tall who weighs 125 pounds will experience the tube as being almost roomy, while another woman of the same height who weighs 175 pounds might have only a few inches on all sides of her body. In recent years, the bore of MRI tubes has increased in diameter to accommodate those who are large in girth, and the weight limitation for most MRIs has recently been increased from 300 pounds to 350 pounds.

For some patients, going into the MRI tube can be a claustrophobic experience. If you find it so, the radiologist can administer a sedative to calm you but not put you to sleep. Some radiologists use Valium given orally or by injection. Injections, because they work instantly, are more predictable and controllable than pills. If you opt to use such sedation, a clip will be placed on one of your fingers to monitor your pulse and oxygenation levels so that you won't be overmedicated.

If you truly think you could not withstand the MRI's confinement, take the time to search for an open-air MRI scanner, which will be easier on you emotionally; however, the quality of the pictures tends not to be as good. Technologists are trying to increase the magnet strength of open MRI scanners, but for now they are between .2 and 1.0 **teslas**, which are units of measuring magnetism. These open scanners are considered to be low-field strength compared to the high-field strength of 1.5 to 3.0 teslas for the closed tubes. The best pictures with the most information come from MRIs with high-field strength scanners of 1.5 teslas or above.

MR Arthrograms

Typically, there are two different MR studies a doctor can order of a hip: a conventional MRI or an MR arthrogram. Current literature says that the radiologist reading your study is going to detect a labral tear with a higher degree of certainty with an MR arthrogram. This special study starts with a routine MRI. Immediately afterward, a radiologist injects a magnetic-like liquid into the hip joint to provide contrast on the MRI. Right after the injection, the patient goes back into the MRI scanner for a few final pictures to end the study. The contrast liquid in the joint outlines the labrum and can show a labral tear that otherwise could go undetected on all other studies including X-ray, CT scan, and the routine MRI. Your doctor may decide an MRA is needed so that you both know everything possible has been done imaging-wise to get information about your hip.

> ### *MR Arthrogram Finds the Labral Tear*
>
> When we look at the MRA, we see bright white areas, which is the contrast liquid I injected into the joint. The entire joint space and the articular cartilage are outlined by this cool-looking white liquid. We can see the contours of the bone more clearly, and we can see the labrum and a little tear where the contrast snuck in. Bingo! There's the tear. Without the contrast, I would have had a very hard time seeing that tear.
>
> —Douglas Brown, MD

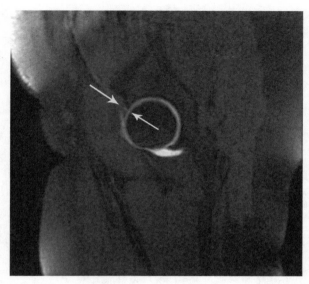

Figure 4-3. The arrows point to a small tear in the labrum found by MR arthrogram.

CT Scans

In the phrase CT scan, or CAT scan, the letters stand for computerized axial tomography. It is a three-dimensional X-ray that shows a full picture of the bones from every possible angle. Like the X-ray, it shows only bone, not the hip's soft tissue structures such as ligaments, tendons, or the labrum.

Like the MRI, a CT scan offers "sliced" views of the body as seen from the front, from the side, and from the top. Thus you can see more detail if you have a complicated bone fracture or if your doctor suspects and is looking for spurs (osteophytes), cysts, or sclerosis. All of these are shown perfectly on a CT scan.

KlapperVision: Think of the socket side of your hip joint as a dome like the United States Capitol building. If the dome is deformed, I want to see what the front, the top, the back, and the sides of the dome look like. An X-ray would give me a view of only the front of the dome, but the CT scan will give me the full picture from every possible angle.

For the CT scan, you'll go into a room with a scanner and lie on a narrow platform. The platform slides into a doughnut-shaped tube that's about two feet deep. Most of your body will be outside the tube except for the portion that is being scanned. The platform will move you through the tube, stopping at specific intervals for each scan. The person taking your scan will be in the control room watching you through a glass window and speaking to you through a microphone. You'll be able to talk to the technician if you're uncomfortable or concerned about anything. Although thirty minutes is usually allotted for the scan, the actual scanning time is approximately fifteen minutes. During that time, you'll need to lie still. You won't feel anything, but you'll hear a whirring sound as the computer moves the X-ray machine around your body. Most patients are relatively comfortable during the procedure.

Future Medical Records

You may eventually have your entire life's medical file, including all the imaging studies and doctors' notes, stored in your phone. If you change doctors, you'll merely give the new doctor the electronic file, and all your data will be instantly available.

—Douglas H. Brown, MD

New Findings on Your Studies

The orthopedic surgeon has to consider many variables when you go to him with hip pain. As a clinician, he'll gather data, put it all together, and narrow it down into certain categories he thinks are most likely. Then, to prove his diagnosis, he will probably start with an X-ray in his own office. If he feels he needs more information, he will send you for the appropriate imaging study.

In this section, we will explain the two new findings that may appear in your studies so you can keep up with the knowledge that is being gained by your doctor and radiologist. Most radiologists who are aware of the new findings of **alpha angle** and **crossover sign** and will put them in their written reports that accompany the studies. Since many patients go to three or more doctors, the radiologist knows they're going to deal with an orthopedic surgeon somewhere down the line who will ask about it. If you see mention of these things on your report, we want you to know what they are. In general, the crossover sign is usually seen on an X-ray, and the alpha angle is a measurement performed on an MRI.

Alpha Angle

Alpha angle is a critical measurement that is drawn digitally onto your MRI by the radiologist. It helps identify **cam** type FAI (see pages 77 and 78). The alpha angle measures how round the head is or if there is extra bone just below the femoral head on the neck that will block easy movement.

KlapperVision: Michael Jordan has a nice silhouette. You can see his shoulders, narrow neck, and wider spherical head. Think of Michael Jordan's neck as the femoral neck and his head as the femoral head. If Michael Jordan wore a scarf around his neck, his silhouette would be different. The scarf would no longer allow you to see the contrast of the narrowness of the neck compared to the size of his head. If it was a thin silk scarf, he might be able to rotate his head from side to side or tilt it one way and then the other. But if the scarf was a thick, dense wool, it may restrict him from making those movements. That's FAI. I can see this cam impingement on a simple X-ray, but I can't tell the degree of the impingement—just as I could tell you from a distance that Michael Jordan was wearing a scarf, but I couldn't tell you how thick it was. If a doctor wants more details about the scarf, you will need to have a CT scan or an MRI.

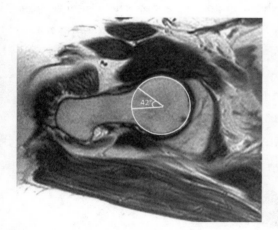

Figure 4-5.
MRI of a 42-degree alpha angle,
no cam impingement.

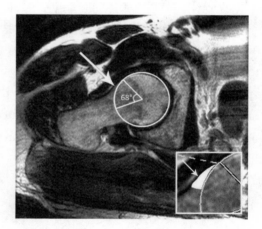

Figure 4-6. MRI of a 68-degree alpha angle.
Large arrow points to cam defect,
more easily seen in inset blow-up.

My opinion is that the alpha angle should be measured solely on an MRI. We're looking for how thick the scarf is, so we need that number. If the alpha angle is 55 degrees or greater, there is cam impingement. If the alpha angle is 54 degrees or below, you can rule out FAI, so your hip pain must be coming from something else.

Crossover Sign

You have probably not thought about the angle of your hip sockets, but they are normally rotated slightly forward. This provides a structural way to fight gravity and create mechanical efficiency.

KlapperVision: Cut an orange in half. Turn one piece to face you as in Photo 4-1A so you see the perfect circle of the orange pulp and the white ring around it. Think of the white ring as the rim of your acetabulum, and imagine the pulp cut out so there's an empty hip socket. Now rotate the orange slightly to the position in Photo 4-1B. As you turn it, the white ring starts looking oblong not circular anymore. You know the orange is still a round sphere, but when it's angled like this, it no longer appears to be a perfect circle. This is what most hips will look like on an X-ray as shown in Figure 4-4. The acetabulum should be angled twenty degrees forward. We call that twenty degrees of **anteversion**. *Ante* means before or in front of you—in this case, facing forward. We can tell how much anteversion there is by how oblong the circle appears. To get a better understanding, review Photos 4-1A, 4-1B, and Figure 4-4.

If your hips are not angled forward but facing directly to the side, we call that a neutral position, as in Photo 4-1C. That may or may not be a problem. **Retroversion** is the opposite of anteversion. *Retro* means going backward. If hip sockets face backward, as in Photo 4-1D, that's called retroversion. It's not always a problem if your hips are retroverted. But each of these findings is important to your doctor if you have a hip problem. If you're having pain and limping, we look to this abnormal anatomy as a potential source of your pain. We factor this in with many other important variables in your history—your work, recreational activities, injury, medications—and try to put together a full picture of your hip problem. Finding retroversion doesn't mean you need surgery. It's just a piece of the puzzle.

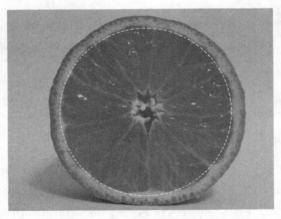

Photo 4-1A. Orange cut in half to represent the acetabulum.
Imagine cutting out the pulp to reproduce a hollow socket.

Picture yourself standing and facing a friend. Think of the oranges as looking at the front of his right hip.

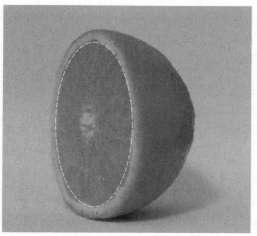

Photo 4-1B. Orange anteverted.

This is the normal angle of your hip socket, slightly facing forward. This oblong appearance of the white line duplicates what we see on the X-ray at the right. Normal anteversion of the hip socket.

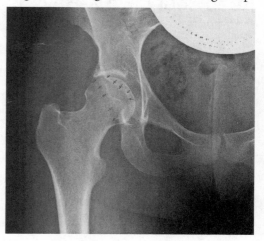

Figure 4-4. Hip anteversion.

Look closely at the dense white rim as outlined by the arrows. The back wall of the socket is on the left. The front wall of the socket is on the right.

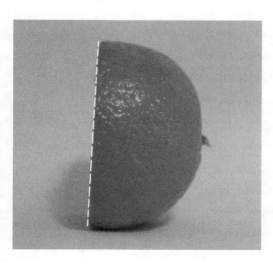

Photo 4-1C. Orange, neutral.

Just as the white line on the orange looks like a straight line, so will the front and back sockets line up to look like a straight line on the X-ray.

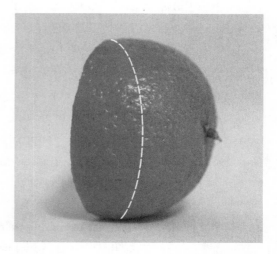

Photo 4-1D. Orange showing retroversion.

The white dotted line is the posterior rim of the socket, which you would see on an X-ray. Notice how this is the reverse of anteversion.

Keep Your Own X-Rays

The world of medicine is changing. So are insurance plans, Medicare, and health maintenance organizations (HMOs). Doctors come in and out of your life. The only constant is you. You need to do everything in your power to keep your current X-rays in your possession and carry them with you when you visit various doctors. If anyone refuses to release your X-rays, respectfully ask for a copy of them. Every patient has the right to a copy of the radiologist's report as well as the images. At the very least, you'll want to have a copy of your pelvis X-ray like the ones in this chapter. Keep all your X-rays together in one electronic folder. If you have plain film in large envelopes, store them in a cool, dark place. Put them flat on top of everything else in a closet or another location where you won't lose them.

Here's an illustration of how important your X-rays can be. Recently I saw two patients who were told they needed hip surgery. They each came to me for a second opinion. One patient was in his late seventies, the other in her early eighties. These patients had had implant surgery over twenty years ago. I could see on each X-ray that the plastic was wearing out on the socket side of the joint. However, neither was having much pain. Still, they were told they had to have a revision of their hip surgeries.

Both of those patients brought along old X-rays. I compared their X-rays from five years before with the new ones and saw no difference. The wear on the plastic had not increased in the past five years. Neither patient was complaining of pain, so I told them both they didn't need surgery but to hang on to their X-rays and that we'd keep an eye on their conditions over time. I wouldn't have been able to make that recommendation without their old X-rays.

Our job in this chapter was to provide you with some basic information about imaging so it won't seem so mysterious. You'll be happy to know that you have learned key buzzwords that both your doctor and your radiologist use when discussing your case. And now, for example, you'll be able to look at your written radiology report to see if an alpha angle was mentioned. You can see if FAI showed up anywhere in the report as a positive or a negative. You can determine if they're having you do an MRI in an open scanner that's low-field strength, less than 1.5 teslas. This knowledge will help you manage your care a little better. You'll be able to ask questions that let the health-care workers around you know that you understand the hip and some of the problems you're facing. You've been empowered.

5

FEMOROACETABULAR IMPINGEMENT

with Daniel Lim, MD

Don't worry about trying to pronounce that complicated name right now. First we want to explain why it's so important.

We used to see either normal hips or hips that were bone-on-bone from osteoarthritis (OA) in need of implant surgery. We hadn't yet learned that there can be a series of steps over many years that are the *cause* of the deterioration of your hip besides osteoarthritis. You may not have OA, but still your hip is worsening, so what's going on? Let's call it the hip's **continuum**. On one end of the continuum is the normal hip; on the other end is a hip that is bone-on-bone. But this is a long continuum—the extremes are quite distinct, but there can be many steps along the way that are almost imperceptibly different from one another.

As we watched time go by and saw a painful hip lose more and more of its cartilage, we didn't yet know there might be a vandal in the house (the hip joint) who was breaking the windows and tearing the place apart. That vandal is femoroacetabular impingement (FAI), and here's the story.

In the 1990s, we thought that perhaps a torn labrum was acting like sandpaper, damaging the cartilage inside the joint, so we cleaned it out arthroscopically. In the early 2000s, a hip arthroscopist in New York started putting stitches into the labrum to repair it. That was groundbreaking at the time. But there was one more step we had to take. We had to protect that labrum from re-injury. Yes, we had cleaned up the vandalized house, but we hadn't chased the vandal away yet. He was still lurking around inside. We were looking for the vandal when surgeons in Switzerland found him inside the hip joint hiding in plain sight. The vandal who was wreaking havoc inside the joint was excess bone on the acetabulum, or on the head/neck junction of the femur. That's FAI. The Swiss doctors had determined a cause-and-effect relationship between a damaged labrum and the deterioration of the hip. And they concluded that abnormal bone development caused the labral damage. They performed open surgeries to remove the bone that was damaging the labrum. Hip arthroscopists in San Francisco said, "Let's do it arthroscopically!" And now hip arthroscopy surgeons both repair the labrum and protect it from re-injury by sculpting away the offending bone.

Femoroacetabular Impingement is quite a mouthful, so let's break it down. *Femoro* refers to your femur or thigh bone; *acetabular* refers to your hip socket, the acetabulum. *Impingement* means to have an effect upon or to strike, especially with a sharp collision. Your femur and your acetabulum are banging into each other, and your labrum is probably being damaged between them with every blow. We call this condition FAI. As you learn the basics about FAI, this knowledge will put you far ahead of many of your peers and possibly even a few of your doctors.

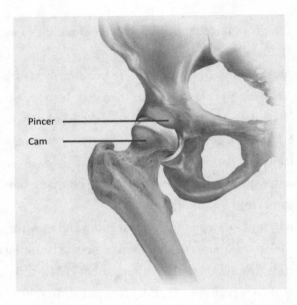

Figure 5-1. FAI, **pincer** and cam type impingements. Pincer: Notice the extra bone on the acetabular rim. This blocks normal motion. Cam: Notice the extra bone at the head/neck junction of the femur. This bump restricts movement.

Let's look at the hip's great mobility as it moves in all three planes of motion. You can move your thigh forward and backward, side to side, and rotate it clockwise and counterclockwise, which is why you can point your toes right or left. The hip's wide range of motion allows you to walk, climb stairs, sit cross-legged, dance, and participate in sports.

In the normal hip joint, the ball of the femur is smooth and regularly shaped, and it fits neatly into the socket. The neck of the femur is normally shaped and free from excess bony growths so the head of the femur has full range of motion in all directions without impinging on the labrum attached to the rim of the acetabulum. A normal hip has full range of motion without any bony impingement. But when the bones of the hip are abnormally shaped, your range of motion is diminished.

You may have known you didn't have as much hip flexibility as other people in your fitness classes or on your sports teams, but until you started having hip pain, you may not have given it much thought. Now you want to know what's causing your pain and what to do about it. If you have FAI, it is the bones colliding, striking, and damaging the nerve-rich labrum that is causing the problem. If you confirm your diagnosis and take action to resolve your pain, you may also be stopping progressive damage to your hip that leads to osteoarthritis. Today we understand how crucial it is that the alignment between the ball and socket be smooth and frictionless.

If you are still growing, we would call your bones skeletally immature. These are the developmental years, and it is during this time that bony abnormalities can develop in your hip joints. Thus FAI isn't a congenital condition—you aren't born with it. Rather it develops between birth and whenever you stop growing. For example, if you're say eighteen or twenty-five, but a coach or a trainer tells you that you lack flexibility in your hips, it's not muscles, ligaments, or tendons. At that age, the soft tissues are fully elastic—the problem is the bone. You may have developed FAI. About 30 percent of the population has FAI, but not all of those people will be bothered by it. Many conduct their lives easily without discomfort, while others experience the pain of a torn labrum and limited movement due to a hip that does not allow full mobility.

Types of Impingement

Impingement can be caused by an enlarged acetabular rim, by a bony growth on the neck of the femur, or by both. Most FAI patients have both. These conditions create a constant banging of the femoral neck onto the rim of the socket, which damages the labrum, the rim of fibrocartilage that runs completely around the acetabulum. Even small irregularities in the bones can eventually cause significant problems over time.

The labrum is a relatively thin rim of fibrocartilage that serves very important functions and when damaged can have significant mechanical consequences. The labrum creates a seal that holds joint fluid inside the hip to serve as a lubricant, creating a smooth, gliding surface. The fluid is also a source of nourishment for articular cartilage, bathing it in nutrients to keep it healthy. Additionally, the seal maintains the negative pressure inside the joint, which is a healthy environment for the cartilage. The labrum is also an extension of the socket that grabs on to the head of the femur and increases the stability of the joint. Figure 5-1 shows both types of impingement, which can cause wear, pain, and ultimately osteoarthritis.

KlapperVision: Picture a car tire moving smoothly within its wheel well. In order to steer that car, there needs to be enough clearance between the tire and the fender so the wheels can turn to the left or right without touching anything. See Figure 5-2A. If the fender is too long or bent out of shape, its rim will scrape against the tire as in Figure 5-3A. If the tire is too large, it will rub against the rim of the fender as in Figure 5-4A. In both situations, there is not enough space for the tire to move freely. Lack of clearance damages the rim of the fender or causes irregular wearing of the tire—or both.

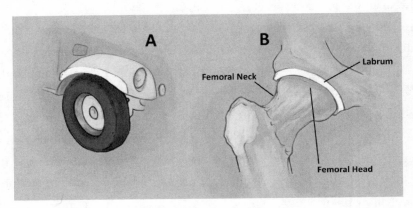

Figure 5-2. A. Compatibility between the tire and the wheel well provides enough clearance to allow the tire to spin easily while being protected inside the wheel well. The white rim of the fender is the equivalent of the labrum. B. The femoral head fits neatly in the socket with no bony impingement from either the acetabulum or the femoral neck.

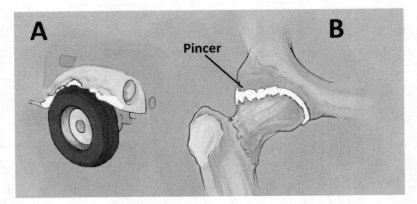

Figure 5-3. A. The rim of the fender is too long for the tire to fit under it with adequate clearance. This lack of clearance scrapes the tire and damages the rim of the fender. B. The acetabulum protrudes too far onto the neck of the femur and causes impact and damage to the labrum.

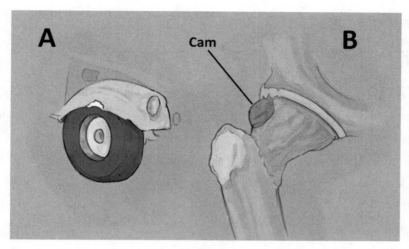

Figure 5-4. A. The tire is too large, causing impingement on both the tire and the rim of the fender. B. The cam defect impinges on the labrum and, over time, tears it and starts to damage the articular cartilage that also attaches to the rim of the acetabulum.

Compare that to your hip joint by thinking of the head of the femur as the tire and the acetabulum as the wheel well. The rim of the fender is the labrum. Not having enough space between the neck of the femur and the rim of the socket causes impact that can injure the labrum. The reverberations of such impact produce damage to the articular cartilage inside the joint, which is the beginning of osteoarthritis.

Pincer Type Impingement

With a pincer type impingement, the problem is the socket. There is extra bone on the rim of the acetabular cup making it disproportionately long and resulting in a socket that is too deep—the ball of the femur cannot move freely within it. The protruding rim of the socket will collide with the neck of the femur. This impacts the soft labrum and eventually causes it to crack, tear, or even calcify to protect itself. Pincer type impingement is usually a congenital problem in which the hip socket is too deep.

Pincer defects are common in middle-aged, active women. They occur through repeated contact between the femoral neck and an over-covered acetabular rim. This results in labral degeneration, often to the point where the labrum ossifies, thus losing its rubbery quality and becoming bonelike.

Cam Type Impingement

With a cam type impingement there is a bony bump at the junction of the head and neck of the femur. This protrusion creates grinding forces that tear the labrum and can tug on and eventually peel away portions of the articular cartilage inside the hip socket. A torn labrum can be a precursor to more serious hip deterioration. The labrum and articular cartilage are both intimately attached to the bony rim of the socket. As the bony protrusion bangs into the labrum, it causes a reverberation from the vibration of the impact, similar to the expanding ripples caused by throwing a rock into a lake. The articular cartilage starts to lift off the bone, delaminates (comes apart in layers), and unglues itself from where it was attached to the subchondral bone. Cam defects, sometimes called lesions, are common in young, active men. In fact, men are twice as likely as women to have a cam type impingement.

Combination of Pincer and Cam Impingements

Pincer and cam impingements seldom occur alone. In fact, the most common type of FAI is the combination of cam and pincer as shown in Figure 5-1 on page 74. There you can see the pincer on the top of the acetabular rim and the cam deformity at the front of the femoral neck.

Symptoms

FAI usually affects active young adults with a gradual onset of pain. The pain is usually in the groin area, although sometimes the pain can occur on the side of the hip. Sharp, stabbing pain may be felt upon twisting, turning, and squatting, but it also can be just a dull ache. The source of the pain can be from a damaged ball, socket, or labrum as well as from muscle spasms in response to this structural damage.

Pain is usually worsened with certain movements, particularly hip flexion (bringing your knee to your chest) and internal rotation. In the early stages of FAI, pain can occur intermittently. If you have FAI, you may experience pain after sitting for long periods or with increased physical activity such as climbing stairs or participating in sports. Sometimes popping sounds can be heard and the hip can "lock" and "catch." These could be signs of damage to the labrum.

Diagnosis

Your doctor will most likely start with the physical exam that we showed in chapter 3. The exam for FAI is shown in Photos 3-3 to 3-5 on page 52. If the physical test is positive for FAI, you would probably have an X-ray and possibly an MRI to rule out or confirm FAI.

If your doctor has given you a diagnosis of FAI, that can be a good thing. If it is caught early enough, you can work in the pool to stop the progression of the problem without surgery. If the impingement must be corrected surgically, the problematic areas on the femoral neck (cam) or rim of the hip socket (pincer) can be reshaped to restore full, pain-free motion. If the labrum has already been torn, new tools and techniques can repair or reconstruct it.

Wilt's Cam Impingement

In 1994, I performed a hip arthroscopy on Wilt Chamberlain, a 7'1" former NBA center. That procedure bought Wilt five years before he needed implant surgery, which he scheduled with me in 1999. Because his hip joint was so much larger than any of the implants made for the general population, we made a computer model of his hip from a CT scan. The implant company created a custom-made implant for him. I still have the model. In the 1990s, we didn't yet know about FAI, but when I look at that anatomical model now, I can see that Wilt had cam type FAI.

—Robert Klapper, MD

See chapter 13 for details about arthroscopic surgery and to see if you might be a candidate. Drawings 13-1 and 13-2 on pages 244 and 245 show how a pincer or cam defect can be removed and the labrum repaired.

6

THE RIGHT TREATMENT

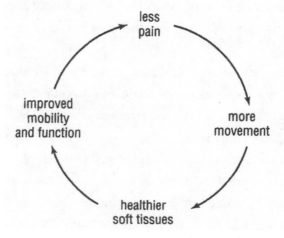

Figure 6-1. Positive Spiral.

Now, with commitment to treatment, you'll enter the Positive Spiral to hip health: less pain leads to more movement, which leads to healthier soft tissues, which leads to improved mobility and function, and so on (see Figure 6-1). Begin by choosing among these conservative treatments that will allow you to enter the Positive Spiral at the point of *less pain*.

Getting Unstuck

I've gathered anecdotal information over the past thirty years from coaching injured athletes in water and on land, and I've reached an interesting conclusion: If a person's pain starts shifting location slightly or the symptoms begin changing, the injury is trying to heal. The body is innately programmed to heal; that's what it does best. When pain is "stuck," unchanging, it seems the healing process is stuck as well. You need to do something to get "unstuck." All of the treatments described in this chapter can start the process.

—Lynda Huey

Aquatic Therapy

Exercising in water—aquatic therapy—can be the best of all pain-reducing treatments. It naturally increases circulation, releases endorphins (the body's painkillers), and stimulates the body's healing mechanisms. Best of all, you can gain all of these benefits without putting any weight on your hip.

Exercising in water is the gentlest, safest way to increase flexibility, increase strength, and gain endurance—in other words, the best way to regain movement, mobility, and function. Further, it is one of only two ways that you can simultaneously make a positive change to multiple joints that are having problems. First, you could take a pill that goes into your stomach, is digested, moves into your bloodstream, and sends its chemicals to every joint in your body. We are not fans of taking pills. The only other treatment that simultaneously affects multiple joints is the pool. In order to perform exercises in the water, you have to use muscles and joints to stand, sit, or balance to do them. You benefit by working these secondary structures that may have become compromised by your bad hip. Thus, if your back or knee has become sore from making compensatory movements to make up for what your hip can't do, you will find the water soothing to them as well, as you work on healing your hip. A thorough description of the unparalleled qualities of water appears in chapter 8.

When you followed the pool program described in chapter 1, you used the water's buoyancy to move your hip through its entire current range of motion. It may have moved more easily in some planes of motion than in others, for example, forward and backward more easily than out to the side. You may have found pain as you stretched your legs wide apart. You gained information about your painful hip that you wrote into your physical history and talked over with your doctor. The longer, more comprehensive pool program in chapter 9 will show you how to progress along the Positive Spiral.

Reduce High-Impact Activities

Reduce the duration of your everyday high-impact activities by climbing fewer stairs, carrying fewer heavy packages, avoiding standing in long lines, doing less taxing yardwork, or walking shorter distances. In addition, modify your sports life: Replace high-impact activities with (in this order) water workouts, bicycling, and elliptical training. If you are a former athlete who can't bear to give up your favorite sport completely, you should use one of these recommended activities for daily fitness and save your sport for soul-satisfying special occasions. See chapter 7 for guidance in setting training limits and for encouragement in making the transition, as thousands of our patients have done, into a newly adopted, nurturing form of exercise.

Benefit Found ONLY in the Water

The most unique advantage of doing a pool program is the **tactile** sensation of the water on your skin. As you move, you feel the pressure of the water gliding over your skin, offering you information. Even if your eyes are closed, you will be able to tell where your leg is or if your hip is bent or straight by feeling the water pressing against your skin. This sense of position is called **proprioception**. The **golgi tendon organs** are sensory receptors in the joints that provide you with information about your body's position, but they can become damaged in the deterioration of your hip. Thus, having lost this sense of body orientation, patients will sometimes say to me, "It feels like my hip is dislocating," which it definitely is not doing. They have lost proprioception. But the water can speak to tiny nerves in the skin. That offers a second pathway to make up for loss of feedback from the damaged golgi tendon organs. By using the secret pathway to proprioception in the water, you can regain your sense of position and stability. By doing our pool program, you can let the water communicate to the deep structures of your hip joint like no other movement form or therapy can. The success we've seen from thousands of patients in the pool is probably due in part to this hidden mechanism— position sense, proprioception training that no other modality offers. Your leg will feel more stable, your hip more secure. That sense can come from strength and flexibility, sure; but it also comes from an improvement in the neuromuscular communication that goes through the damaged sensors in the joint that are aided by the tactile touching of the water on the skin.

—Robert Klapper, MD

Wear Impact-Absorbing Shoes

The harder your shoes, the more impact you are transmitting to all your weight-bearing joints, including your hip. That translates to more trauma to the articular cartilage surfaces and more erosion. Wear the highly cushioned athletic shoes made for runners. That may not be realistic all the time given the demands and dress codes of your workplace, but wear them whenever you can.

Cortisone Injections

It is well known in the medical community that injecting cortisone into a joint damages the surfaces of the vital articular cartilages in that joint. Yes, cortisone is a miraculous anti-inflammatory that knocks out pain and swelling (sometimes temporarily, sometimes forever), but it may damage working surfaces of the joint and can leave behind—to linger forever in your joint—the gritty, powdery substance found in some cortisone preparations. Repeated injections into a joint literally "spoil" that joint. Doctors know that, but we look at the trade-off.

Yes, I've injected cortisone into a hip on exceptional occasions: a desperate patient going to Italy for the first time and couldn't exchange his plane tickets; a distraught mother with debilitating pain who wanted to walk down the aisle at her daughter's wedding. In both cases I made sure the patient understood the risk, and I made the shot available.

—Robert Klapper, MD

Lose Weight

Your hip is the largest of your weight-bearing joints. Every time you take a step, you load your hip with more than three times your body weight, so if you weigh 150 pounds, your hip has to support over 450 pounds with each step. Every pound you gain means more than three pounds of pressure placed on your hip with each step. Conversely, if you were to lose ten pounds, you would eliminate thirty pounds of pressure that your hip must bear. *Now is the time to lose weight by dieting and starting a low-impact exercise program.* Don't think you can keep eating the same and just increase your exercise. You have a sore hip, and that needs protecting. You can't exercise yourself into shape with a bad diet. Calories are about 95 percent of the solution. Always put the priority on reducing your food intake—that's the way to lose weight no matter what's changing in your world of exercise.

Weight Loss Tips

Several times in my life, I've added extra pounds and couldn't seem to control my eating. I've never been more than ten pounds overweight, but that's a lot on a 5'3" frame. I have always fought my way back to my ideal weight. Here are my tried-and-true tips to start the weight-loss process:

1. Have some protein for breakfast. It doesn't have to be eggs or a typical breakfast food. I've relied on a protein shake every morning for the past three decades. Find a breakfast that will make you feel stable—not hungry and not thinking about food for at least three hours.
2. When you've finished eating, brush your teeth so you won't crave more.
3. No recreational eating. Prescribe nutritional food for yourself.
4. No seconds. One portion of food at a meal is plenty.
5. Weigh yourself at the same time every morning. If your weight has gone up, you have to do better that day. If it has gone down, congratulate yourself and gain encouragement from that.
6. Don't buy items for which you have a weakness. If you don't have them in the house, you can't eat them.
7. Let fruit satisfy your sweet tooth. Eat watermelon, grapes, berries, or peaches instead of muffins, cake, or brownies. A cake might look good, but picture it as many heaping tablespoons of sugar going into your body.

8. Negotiate with yourself. Simply *must* have that one special thing to eat right now? Commit to swapping it with something else in your food plan for the day and stick to it. Don't eat both.

9. Ask yourself if you're hungry before you eat anything. Don't eat when you're not hungry.

10. Drink a glass of water when you feel tired or start to think about snacking. It's possible you are dehydrated rather than hungry, and water will give your tissues and joints what they need.

11. Strong discipline deserves a reward. Every once in a while, treat yourself to a special food that you would otherwise avoid—and enjoy it!

—Lynda Huey

There's no mystery about losing weight. You have to increase your exercise and cut down on your eating. If you don't think you can manage this alone, get whatever help you need. Join a low-impact exercise program or hire a personal trainer to motivate you to work out consistently. Choose one of the many weight-loss organizations that are available. Create an exercise/food management program that you're comfortable with so you'll stick with it and really take off some fat. Your hip is at risk, so get serious. If you've tried to lose weight many times and failed, consult with your internist or a nutritionist.

Ice

Ice is the most underrecognized of all painkillers. It needs no prescription, is easy to apply, and is quick to begin working—and it's free. Applying ice to your sore hip reduces blood flow, slows nerve conduction, and elevates your pain threshold. Because it cuts your pain, it reduces your need for pain medication. Keep in mind that ice treats only the tissues closest to the skin—it works well in reducing muscular pain, tendinitis, and bursitis, but it won't reduce pain or swelling deep inside your hip joint.

Fill a large plastic freezer bag with ice cubes and place it on the part of your hip where you feel pain. If your skin is particularly sensitive, put a thin cloth between the ice bag and your skin. Leave the ice bag in place for ten to fifteen minutes, but check your skin under the ice several times to make sure your skin isn't being burned by the ice. When you remove the ice, wrap a dry towel around the cold skin, and enjoy the "thawing" sensation. If your hip hurts in more than one place, move the ice to another sore spot for another ten to fifteen minutes.

> ### A Free Miracle
>
> Ice is the closest you can come to a free miracle. It is nature's best anti-inflammatory. It can knock out pain and speed the healing of many injuries. Look at ice as a quiet but powerful cure. I swear by it and advise all those I work with to ice after leaving the pool.
>
> —Lynda Huey

If you become a devoted fan of ice, you'll want to give your hip an ice massage. Fill a Styrofoam cup with water and put it in the freezer. Once frozen, peel down the Styrofoam until about an inch of ice is exposed. What's left of the cup becomes a "handle" for this ice-massage device. Begin making circular or back-and-forth motions with the ice cup on the sore areas of your hip. When your skin turns pink and feels numb, wrap your hip in a dry towel.

For convenience and adjustable compression as well as complete mobility, the reusable ACE Multi-Purpose Wrap can be used instead of ice bags. The ACE system consists of a freezable gel pack that fits into an insulated Neoprene-blend encasement with stretchy Velcro straps to wrap around your body. The straps stay snugly around you, holding the gel pack in the most desirable position over your hip, buttock, or groin. With the ACE wrap firmly in place, you can continue your daily activities at home or at work with none of the mess of ice bags. The gel pack can also go in the microwave and be heated to offer contrast treatments, which are discussed in the following section. Whether the gel pack is used frozen for cold treatment or microwaved for heat treatment, the insulation of the Neoprene wrap maintains the proper therapeutic temperature throughout each treatment.

Contrast Ice and Heat

Ice decreases cell metabolism and increases tissue stiffness. Heat increases cell metabolism and decreases tissue stiffness. Both ice and heat decrease pain. Use ice as the only treatment for the first forty-eight hours if you have a sudden or **acute** injury to the hip. If the hip problem is considered **chronic**, both ice and heat can be used. Apply heat. Follow it immediately with ice. Go back and forth several times: heat, ice, heat, ice—this alternation is called contrast ice and heat. Heat causes **vasodilation**, an increase of blood supply to the area, then ice brings about **vasoconstriction**, a decrease in the blood supply. These contrast treatments confuse the body by bombarding it with stimulants that are opposites. The confusion causes an escalated response and a tremendous amount of circulation and healing to the area.

At home, use a heating pad or place your ACE gel pack in the microwave for one minute to create a hot pack. Wrap the hot gel pack in a thin towel to prevent burning. After fifteen minutes, switch to ten minutes of ice. As the ice treatment begins, you may feel a deepening of the pain, an aching from the cold. Then as the numbing occurs, virtually all deep pain is gone. When the heat is applied again, the cold tissues go through a "thawing" sensation that most people find pleasurable. Finish your contrast treatment with ten minutes of ice. Hot showers, baths, hot tubs, and cold pools are also appropriate contrast treatments for pain management. In the hot tub, sit in a position that allows the jet stream to flow directly toward the sore area of your hip.

Physical Therapy

Physical therapists are considered movement specialists. They look at your movement patterns, body alignment, and treatment goals as they develop a rehabilitation plan to help you restore or maintain strength, mobility, and function. Physical therapists offer various treatments, including gait training, postural training, therapeutic exercise, and advanced manual techniques such as joint and soft tissue mobilization. They will use modalities such as ultrasound or electrotherapy when needed to reduce your pain, swelling, or both, and they will teach you a home exercise program to help you become independent in managing your hip problem. (See chapters 11 and 12 for more details about physical therapy.)

Gait training. Proper gait, walking, is essential in maintaining upright posture, preventing falls, and performing normal activities of daily living. The therapist will evaluate all phases of your gait, find what needs correcting, and help you improve the way you walk and balance.

Postural training. In order to develop strength, power, speed, and balance in all activities of your life, you must have proper posture. This isn't cosmetic; it's functional. Without good posture, you can't reach your full potential in any activity. Good posture reduces your risk of injury just as bad posture increases that risk. Therapists will help you strengthen your postural muscles and balance the strength in key **core muscles** that contribute to a smoother-functioning hip.

Therapeutic exercise. By using functional activities such as bending, lifting, carrying, reaching, catching, and overhead activities, therapists help you train your body for the activities you perform in daily life. Your exercises will be chosen to address a loss or restriction of mobility, strength, balance, or coordination. Chapter 11 explains some of the physical principles behind the stretching and strengthening land program in chapter 12.

Advanced manual therapy techniques. By elongating and manipulating soft tissues beyond their restrictions, the therapist relieves muscle spasms, softens tight and inflamed tendons and connective tissue, increases blood flow, and generally aids in restoring health and function to your hip. When the therapist's hands are applying pressure to the tissues, you will often feel increased pain, but as soon as the pressure is released, your tissues will feel more mobile and less painful. When a therapist mobilizes a hip joint, she applies skilled passive movement directly to the joint in order to increase mobility and decrease pain.

Ultrasound. Therapeutic ultrasound mechanically vibrates tissues at an extremely high frequency. This micromassage raises the tissue's temperature through friction, which improves circulation, resulting in increased cellular metabolism, thus accelerating the healing process. Ultrasound is applied to the skin through a water-based gel. Medications can be added to the gel so that the ultrasound drives the medicine through the skin into the underlying tissues. When ultrasound is used in this way, it is called **phonophoresis.**

Electrotherapy. Research has shown that electrotherapy works well in pain management. It also helps improve local blood flow, and it can accelerate the rate at which the body absorbs swelling. It can improve the range of joint mobility and restore the integrity of connective tissue. (The pain-relieving device called a TENS unit is most likely borrowing technology learned from acupuncture and bringing it to Western medicine.)

Modalities

When doctors or physical therapists speak of using a modality, they are referring to the application of a therapeutic agent. These therapeutic agents can be anything from ice to heat to electrotherapy. They are all modalities, and they help arouse the body's natural healing forces while decreasing pain and swelling. While they can make you feel better, they are strictly an adjunct to the exercises that are the true heart of your program. Modalities can be a temporary solution to pain; improved strength and flexibility are the long-term solutions.

Chiropractic

Chiropractic searches out the root of imbalance and treats your whole body, even if it seems you have solely a hip problem. Since all the joints move in relation to one another, your hip may be affected by musculoskeletal imbalances in other areas of your body. Chiropractic treatment can help restore structural balance by addressing posture, spinal alignment, pelvic and lower back stability, and shoulder and hip range of motion, as well as knee, ankle, and foot conditions that could be affecting the hip.

If your hip has been painful for a long time, you may have begun to compensate for limited hip motion by limping, leaning, twisting, or moving your pelvis. Such compensatory movements can create aches and pains in your lower back, your knees, and elsewhere. Chiropractors can help identify and correct these imbalances and abnormal movements to help you return to normal function. Many chiropractors perform manipulations that can free joint and nerve restrictions that cause hip pain.

It is the good chiropractor who recognizes the connection between the lower back and the hip and can correctly diagnose that when limited motion persists despite treatment, it's time for you to seek the advice of an orthopedic surgeon.

Pilates

Pilates is a fitness system developed by Joseph Pilates, who was born in Germany and lived in England before coming to New York City around 1925. He believed that lifestyle, bad posture, and inefficient breathing lay at the root of poor health. Over many years, he devised a series of exercises and training techniques and engineered all the equipment he needed to teach his methods properly. Well-known dancers such as George Balanchine and Martha Graham became devotees of his techniques and regularly sent their professional dancers to the Pilates gym on 8th Avenue for training and rehabilitation. Joseph Pilates had been a sickly child, so he worked his whole life to create exercises designed to improve posture, strength, stability, and mobility as well as repair imbalances and reduce stress while also developing long, lean muscles without bulk. The ballerinas learned that as they became stronger, they also had the ability to move more freely. Pilates emphasized the mind-body connection and instructed them on precise breathing techniques that gave them the strength to withstand a difficult performance. His exercises were taught on machines he built called the Reformer, the Cadillac, and the Trapeze Table. His theory of the body's "powerhouse" is quite similar to today's concept of "core strength."

The popularity of Pilates is increasing worldwide both in fitness and rehabilitation programs. A decade ago it was practiced by five thousand people; today that number has grown to over five million in the United States alone.

Avoid Pain When Doing Pilates

When doing Pilates, pay close attention to your body's reaction to each position. You or your instructor may need to modify certain body positions to avoid triggering hip pain. Any movement that requires you to spread your legs wider than hip-width apart or to bend deeply at the hip should be avoided. Avoid stretches that require lying on your side if that causes you pain. Exercises such as side-lying leg lifts press your hip bone into the mat, which could cause pain in or around the joint. Also avoid stretches that ask you to bring your knee toward your chest past hip level or that require you to move your leg across your body instead of stopping at the midline.

Beginners should start with mat Pilates, which teaches a series of specialized calisthenics exercises to be performed on the floor rather than on the Reformer. By starting on the mat first, you can stretch your muscles and strengthen your abdominals as you learn to focus on proper placement of your hips. If you progress onto the Reformer or the Cadillac, don't use the straps or springs, and keep your feet less than hip-width apart. Since Joseph Pilates created his machines and exercises for rehabilitation of patients in hospitals, they can be very beneficial. But you should not attempt to perform these Pilates machine exercises by yourself. A qualified Pilates instructor will teach you proper technique, alignment, and breathing as well as modifications to accommodate the limitations of your hip.

—LaReine Chabut, author and certified Pilates instructor

Yoga

The practice of therapeutic yoga offers more than just a series of sustained stretches—it integrates your breath with the movements you make and the positions you hold, giving you increased body awareness. Yoga postures and movements are coordinated with slow, deep breathing. Since the breathing muscles are the same muscles as the postural core muscles, learning to coordinate your breath with the movement increases both your postural and breathing efficiency while also helping to reduce muscular tension and pain.

If you have limited range of motion in your hip but your X-rays show no mechanical reason for the lack of movement, yoga can be an effective method for relieving your pain and gaining strength and flexibility. As you relax deeply into each sustained stretch, you may discover that the tightness around your hip gradually releases and gives you more movement in every plane.

Yoga Classes

Choose your yoga class carefully. You'll find a vast array of classes, but many of these have become westernized "workouts." You want a class that balances stretching and strengthening—one that alternates activity with relaxation. Your intent is to relieve pain, not stress an already troubled hip joint. Many group yoga classes have become extremely athletic and may involve hands-on adjustments of your form by the instructor, which can force your body into painful positions not helpful to your condition. If you are a beginner, be very cautious about participating in these classes. Look for beginning classes or therapeutically oriented classes taught by instructors who know how to modify exercises for those with hip problems. Beware of the following alignment cues that could hurt your hip: "square your hips," or "fold from the hips." Learn to listen to your own body so that you can differentiate joint pain (which is telling you to stop) from the discomfort of stretching and using muscles in a new way.

—Leslie Kaminoff, author of *Yoga Anatomy*

Acupuncture

Acupuncture has been a standard medical practice for thousands of years in Asia as part of traditional Chinese medicine. In 1997, the National Institutes of Health (NIH) declared there is clear evidence that acupuncture is an effective modality. Acupuncturists insert thin needles through the skin at specific points on the body to relieve pain and stimulate the body's natural healing systems. It has been in use in Western society for decades. Health-care practitioners point to the fact that acupuncture is simple and often works. It has few side effects or complications, and the cost is low. For these reasons, it can be a good alternative treatment to consider.

Gene Therapy and the Latest Research

A **gene** is a portion of a DNA molecule that serves as the basic unit of heredity. Genes are the blueprint for making you who you are. Genes tell every cell of your body what to do and when to do it. Some genes are turned "on" so that they begin working, and others are turned "off," doing nothing. Scientists continue to learn more and more about each specific gene and the factors that contribute to turning a gene on or off.

If you have osteoarthritis, and if your mother or father had it before you, it's likely you inherited the gene that causes the development of OA. But what if that gene could be located and turned off permanently? That's the goal of genetic research and the hope of millions of parents who wish not to pass along their diseases to their children.

Gene therapy thus targets the disease process of any condition rather than the symptoms. For instance, we know that at least 50 percent of osteoarthritis cases are genetic in source, so we want to target the genetic process that leads to the degeneration of cartilage rather than simply work to alleviate the pain and inflammation that comes from such degeneration.

The most common form of gene therapy replaces an abnormal gene with a normal gene, one that does not carry the command to break down cartilage. Other approaches work to repair an abnormal gene or alter the degree to which a gene is turned on or turned off. Think of fighting back Father Time and all the manifestations of degeneration. Father Time dries us out—our heart valves, the lenses in our eyes, the articular cartilage in our joints, and the fibrocartilage in the labrum, meniscus, and disks of the spine. We're trying to find a way to put those On/Off switches in our genes onto a dimmer switch. The end result would be the same, but we're hoping that gene therapy can slow down the process. Wouldn't it be vastly better if you could get forty more years out of your problematic hip instead of only ten, twenty, or thirty?

Nothing in Life is Without Side Effects

When you read something about a new treatment that sounds too good to be true, be skeptical. It's exciting to look to the future and hope that we can change at a cellular level how our bodies are affected by disease. But tread carefully. Yes, we can make cells grow, but cells that continue to grow and don't stop are called cancer. Some clinical trials are trying to find out if we can repair a pothole in cartilage. Can we take cells and fill in the holes and the cracks that are developing in the cartilage? Do the new cells fill up to the surface and stop there, flush with the rest of the cartilage? Or does the injected material keep growing and become a bump in the cartilage or worse?

We would love to tell you about a new pill or injection that will change the course of the arthritic or traumatic condition of your hip. There are many promising treatments on the horizon, such as injections of Interleukin 1RA, which proponents say counteracts the inflammation and degenerative process of OA. But it's too early; the answer simply isn't here yet.

For now, we're choosing to remain holistic and go back to our mission statement: We want to empower you to ask the right questions so you don't end up with hip surgery. Before you go under the knife, take three months. See if you can regain a smoothly functioning hip with our beautiful pool program. Stop damaging your hip by replacing your abusive exercise routines with nurturing ones. If, after three months you can honestly say you're not feeling better, then you should consider surgery—but not before.

—Robert Klapper, MD

So far, OA is irreversible and incurable, and we have not yet developed a biological replacement for articular cartilage. But research is underway. Clinical studies are being performed on the complex problem of repairing damaged cartilage. For each study, three ingredients come into play. First, there must be cartilage cells or **stem cells** that are capable of giving rise to an indefinite number of more cells of the same type. Second, **scaffolding** has to exist to keep the cells inside a cartilage defect and act as a support for inducing cartilage formation. Third, **growth factors** must be added to the mix, which stimulate cellular function, growth, and rate of **proliferation**. The growth factors most often used in this research are **platelet-rich plasma (PRP)** and **bone marrow cell concentrate (BMCC)**. These components are being tried in various combinations, and one day we may have the answer. For now, this research is in its infancy. It's a good step so far.

Learning About the Future with a Salamander?

Research that could potentially bring a solution for damaged cartilage is taking place at Harvard University and grew out of their stem-cell research program. They are looking at how a salamander can completely regrow a limb when it is lost. Unlike humans, salamanders do not create scar tissue. In fact, if a salamander's cut leg is sutured closed, it will not regenerate. There appears to be a signal in the salamander's skin that stimulates the regrowth of limbs. This may mean that the step where humans make a scar is stopping other regenerative growth processes that could be more complete like a salamander's. This research may lead to clues for the future—perhaps we may find a way in which cartilage becomes able to regenerate its own natural structure.

7

WIN-WIN: PREVENTION OR PREHAB

The Fountain of Youth Is in the Fountain

Thousands of people have followed our pool program and have actually postponed or prevented surgery. The value of the water program is truly beyond any drug that will ever be invented. It works in ways we don't yet fully understand—and it always surprises people with its effectiveness. As the water touches your skin, it increases your sense of position with feedback to your brain called **proprioception**. In water you'll find less impact yet more resistance to strengthen the muscles around your hip.

—Robert Klapper, MD

Just as in the world of business, we like to talk about a win-win situation. Working to prevent hip surgery can create several wins for you. The ultimate win, of course, is that you follow the programs in this book, relieve your hip pain and dysfunction, and never need hip surgery of any kind. But there are several other possible wins. After several months of doing our pool program, you are likely to realize you're in great shape, so you keep the water at the center of your lifelong fitness plan. It may turn out that you've postponed the need for hip surgery by five or ten years. That's significant because technology keeps improving, and the surgery of the future will no doubt be superior and easier. But the other win is that even if you find yourself eventually scheduling a surgery, you will have become much stronger and able to bounce back more quickly.

Let's say you come to our pool. When we first see you, we won't be certain which path you will be on: Will you be avoiding the surgery? Postponing it? Doing a **prehab** program that will get you stronger before surgery? As we begin, it doesn't matter. We just get started with our highly successful pool program—*always* with the intention of preventing surgery. About a month into the program, we expect to see improvement, first in pain reduction, then in improved range of motion, strength, and flexibility. We modify our expectations and plan for the future based on the results we see.

You can do the same. Just start! Do the work and see where it takes you. Don't be impatient. It might take up to a month before you start feeling improvement. Don't give up too soon! You may be one of the lucky ones who regains good function and strength in your hip, and even though your X-ray or MRI hasn't changed, you are out of pain and no longer considering surgery. Or you may not be quite that lucky, but you're starting to get a good feeling about your pool program, and you suspect that you don't have to rush right into the operating room. This chapter is here to help guide you through the most likely scenarios you will face as you take responsibility for your hip and systematically research and test your options.

Consider the story of a forty-seven-year-old man who, literally overnight, developed pain in both hips. His orthopedic surgeon took X-rays and MRIs and told him he needed implant surgery. By his own acknowledgment this patient had been a couch potato for ten years preceding the diagnosis. He'd lost strength and flexibility from inactivity; so to prepare for surgery, he followed the pool program in chapter 9 twice a week for eight weeks. At the end of that time he was walking without his cane, with no pain in either hip.

By exercising, he had rejuvenated the blood vessels to his muscles and improved his muscle tone. Exercise had caused a hormonal cascade: chemicals stimulated the body to make blood vessels, which increased blood supply to the hip area. The patient earned himself a reprieve from surgery. He bought time. If his hips trouble him again in six months or in a year or two, if the pool program doesn't work for him the next time, then he can consult his surgeon and reschedule the operation. It's not uncommon for a hip-implant patient to have several such surgeries in a lifetime, so the longer he can put off the first one, the less likely he'll need the second.

Review Your Activities

As you work toward *not* having hip surgery, you'll want to do everything you can to stack the odds in your favor. You want to eliminate everything that harms your hip and causes pain while you consistently do the things that help your hip and reduce your pain. If you have been exercising regularly, it may have been in an activity that has been doing damage to your hips. The extreme turn-out performed by ballet dancers takes their hips continually into punishing positions. Gymnasts repeatedly push their hips into wide ranges of motion. Kickboxers and other martial artists not only kick into wildly extreme ranges of motion with their hips, they do so against resistance and the sudden stop of impact. You may not be doing anything so dramatic as these types of activities, but perhaps you noticed that after you finished a tennis match or a five-mile hike your hip started hurting. Yet you did the same thing the next day because that's your favorite sport. It's the one you love. You did it in spite of the growing pain in your hip. But now you know you won't be able to tolerate the pain again tomorrow.

A Wake-Up Call

If hip pain has interrupted your regular workouts, consider it a wake-up call. Use this time to learn to read your body's monitoring systems and learn to interpret the messages your body sends you with its pain signals. Always move away from activities that cause pain and toward those that do not. Don't just take anti-inflammatories and "push through" the pain.

Exercise comes in two flavors: **nurturing** and **abusive**. The sports that people love most—running, basketball, tennis, skiing, racquetball, and football—abuse the body's weight-bearing joints, whereas pool exercise, bicycling, elliptical machines, Tai Chi, mat Pilates, and therapeutic yoga remove impact from the weight-bearing joints and are therefore nurturing. Most people don't consider the abusiveness of their exercise routines until pain or physical limitation strikes. At that point, they pay attention. Our hope is that you'll begin nurturing exercises on a regular basis. By using safe forms of exercise most of the time to maintain and enhance fitness, you may be able to participate in your beloved sports and activities on an occasional basis for years to come.

Take a two-pronged approach to solving your hip problem. First, critically look at your lifestyle, your play, and your family commitments, and delete what we believe is abusive exercise. Do you have a sedentary job? After work do you go to the gym, overtrain, and hurt yourself? Your body doesn't appreciate that. You need to reduce or delete the offensive exercises that may be fun but are damaging your hip.

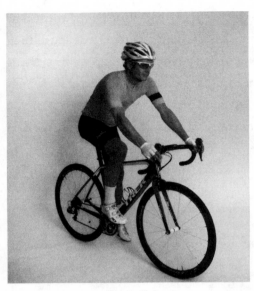

Photo 7-1.

If you don't have access to a pool, try our next favorite nurturing activity: bicycling.

Many people with sore hips have never exercised. Others haven't exercised in years or have exercised far too little. Now is the time to realize that you must take responsibility for your hips and get them moving again. Learn what your body responds to without discomfort. You may love gliding through water, but find that a pool's chlorine irritates your skin. You may love bicycling, but discover that the biking movement causes a pinching feeling in the front of your hip. Try the Pilates and yoga options in chapter 6 or discover other activities of your own choosing. A friend might invite you to her favorite Zumba class, an interval-style class set to Latin rhythm dance music that is exercise in disguise. Or you may learn that you enjoy body boarding, and your hip feels terrific when you get out of the ocean. It's up to you to find what fits your lifestyle, your personal tastes, and most important what your hip *likes*. You might get carried away in a new sport but find that your hip aches terribly that night. Your hip gets the final vote. As much as you like that activity, cross that one off your list.

Pain is your guide. Stop harmful activities when your body whispers to you with a slight pain. Don't wait for your body to shout at you. By then it is too late.

Successful Transition to Your Nurturing Activity

You've grown to love certain sports and activities throughout your lifetime because these activities give you the most satisfaction and pleasure. You've gotten good at the details of your game or fitness regimen, and it won't be easy to walk away from that vital part of your life. You will go through a transition time while your mind and body adapt to the new movements and environments. Perhaps you have always been an outdoor person, and now you're considering an indoor class at the gym. It may take weeks before you will feel the same satisfaction in your new yoga or Pilates regimen. Or if a lifetime of successful tennis has become part of your identity, it may take some time for you to feel the same about another activity.

Like anything new, it takes a while for your mind to become part of the new activity. It takes time before your body begins performing the new skills automatically. Remind yourself that in order to stop hurting your hips, you are making a lifelong change in your fitness routine—then give yourself whatever time that change is going to take.

Do Six Workouts Before Evaluating

Some people get frustrated when they don't see immediate progress. When I work with elite athletes who are coming back after injury, I always tell them, "Just put your head down and do six workouts. Don't look up until we've finished them. Then we'll see how you're doing." Apply this same logic to your new program, especially if you are moving from abusive to nurturing activities. Do six pool or bicycling workouts without judging anything. Once you feel that you're mastering the new skills and creating the specific strength needed, you'll feel an increase in your affinity for your new activity. Soon you'll be finding mental meaning and inner purpose in your physical movements just as you did with your previous activities.

—Lynda Huey

A former elite distance runner had to stop running due to hip pain. She had two small children to keep her from dropping into despair, but she missed running terribly. She came to our pool and started with deep-water running and walking in order to have no weight bearing whatsoever. Her hip pain began to subside—and her enjoyment of deep-water running began to rise. After six weeks in deep water, she made the transition to running and jumping exercises in chest-deep water. She was quite astonished at how much pleasure she felt while running high-intensity intervals with her feet on the bottom of the pool. It *almost* felt like running! She had successfully made the transition from a high-impact sport that hurt her hip to a satisfying but much lower-impact activity that was therapeutic for her hip.

The Decades of Your Life

As we age, most of us need glasses to read. Even if we didn't need glasses before, Father Time is now in our eyes. So we modify our vision with glasses. And we must make other changes out of respect for Father Time as we move from one decade to another.

How to Agercise: How to Exercise for Your Age

Athletes		Abusive	Nurturing
20-30	Enjoy three or more abusive activities	3+	
30-40	Enjoy three or more abusive activities	3+	
40-50	Two abusive activities	2	
50-60	Two abusive activities	2	
60-70	One sport if you begin to relinquish the other abusive ones	1	2
70+	Integrating more nurturing exercises into the routine	0	2+

Others		Abusive	Nurturing
20-30	Do everything you want	3+	
30-40	One or two abusive exercises	1 - 2	
40-50	Decade of Delete—introduce more nurturing activities to combat the abusive ones	2	2
50-60	One abusive exercise, but only if you do two parts nurturing to one part abuse	1	2
60-70	Delete the abuse	0	2
70+	Stick with the pool, Tai chi, yoga, Pilates, and stationary bicycling	0	2+

Figure 7-1. How to Agercise. See page 99 for lists of abusive and nurturing activities.

HEAL YOUR HIPS

The physical ability and function that you may have at any age is very wide ranging. Let's start with the athletes. In your twenties, your body is so resilient that you can enjoy three or more abusive activities without negative consequences. Maybe you go for runs every morning, then play basketball two nights a week and volleyball and football on the weekends. True athletes, people whose bodies are strong, flexible, well balanced, and coordinated, can often continue with such activities into their thirties or even their forties. If you are one of these athletes, and if you escaped major injury in your sports career, you may be able to continue with two abusive activities throughout your forties, possibly into your fifties. But let pain be your guide. It might be time to learn stand-up paddle boarding, kayaking, body boarding, or another activity that uses your upper body more than your lower body.

Since you built good form and strong muscles for your activities, you can often continue into your sixties and seventies to enjoy one sport if you begin to relinquish the other abusive ones. It's time to start alternating your road running with your pool running, or your basketball playing with your bicycling. After age seventy, it's no longer about competition; it's about holding on to as much strength as you can. It's time to start taking the long view—planning how to be active the rest of your life. It means integrating more nurturing exercises into your routine every week.

Baby Boomers Push the Limits

Nearly everyone knows someone who is in his or her sixties or seventies and is superfit. These are the Baby Boomers saying, "No! We won't stop our favorite activities just because we're older." As a Boomer myself, I know many of these superfit people who continue to move gracefully. All of us who continue to thrive athletically have maintained good body weight, get enough sleep, and watch what we eat. If we had small injuries in our athletic careers (hamstring strains, ankle sprains, rotator cuff strains, knee sprains), we systematically and painstakingly did the rehab to return to our full, former levels of function. And we switched sports any time an injury told us to. If you wish to be a superfit seventy-year-old, follow our lead. **Don't let a small injury knock you down a notch and keep you there. Fight your way back to make a full comeback every time.** And start your nurturing exercises now!

—Lynda Huey

Let's say you would call yourself a Regular Joe or Joan. When you are between the ages of twenty and thirty, you have our permission to do everything you want. You're going to heal quickly from a pulled muscle, from a fracture, from straining or tearing this or that. Go for it! When you are in your thirties and get close to forty, you need to begin recognizing that certain exercises abuse your body. You enjoy doing them, but they are abusive. Between thirty and forty, we're asking you to use common sense and start asking yourself some questions, such as, "Should I really be doing this today?" This decade still allows you to have one or two abusive exercises, but it's also time to start thinking about a long-term plan. When you turn forty, you have entered the Decade of Delete. You don't have to delete all of your sports. But you must start introducing more nurturing activities to combat the abusive ones. We would allow you to have two abusive exercises if you add two nurturing ones. Spend time on the bike and in the pool or doing another nurturing exercise of your choice.

Pain Is Your Friend

That's right, pain is your friend. It's what makes us unique. Your training partner may be able to perform an activity with no pain, but you can't. The pain is telling you that you're built differently and that you're hurting yourself with the same movements that your friend can tolerate. Our culture tells us to get rid of the pain with anti-inflammatories or painkillers. The people who do that are the ones I see in my office every week who took those drugs so they could go to the gym and further abuse their bodies without the natural feedback of pain telling them they were hurting themselves. Now they need me to repair their hips surgically because they waited too long to come see me and kept doing further damage. You can listen to the pain, modify your activity, and not go that route.

—Robert Klapper, MD

If you're already in your forties and didn't build a strong body in your youth, you should be participating in no more than one abusive activity that you love to do—but not daily. On the other days, you can begin making up for lost time by giving yourself the gift of fitness using nurturing activities. By cross-training in a pool, on a bike, or on an elliptical machine, you will not only add new layers of strength and flexibility, but you will also be "rationing" the sport you love so that you can enjoy it over many more years. Once you turn fifty, you're allowed only one abusive exercise, but only if you do two parts nurturing to one part abuse. For example, do a bike workout on Monday, a pool workout on Tuesday, then go for a run on Wednesday. When you turn sixty, you have to delete the abuse. It's just not good for you. When you turn seventy, stick with the pool, Tai chi, yoga, Pilates, and stationary bicycling.

Take Responsibility for Your Hip

Readers often email us asking us what to do next. They've seen one or more orthopedic surgeons, sometimes with conflicting opinions of what to do; they've had X-rays and MRIs; and they turn to the Internet looking for an alternative to surgery. They find this book, which offers many treatment options and ideas to delay or prevent hip surgery.

You're reading this book, but now what do you do?

Use the information in this chapter to help plan your next step. Keep reading. In the next few pages, you will learn how to design your own pool/land program, or a land-only program. By now you know that we strongly urge you to make whatever effort you must to gain access to a pool, especially one with deep water. That's where the magic happens. But we're realistic. We know some of you live too far from a pool, can't tolerate pool chemicals, or are simply stuck at home some days. The land-only program is for you.

Do your program three to five times a week. Be disciplined; don't miss days.

Don't worry about what's next until you've been doing your rehab program for at least three months. By then you'll have an idea if you're doing a prevention program or a prehab program. A caution: Don't leap to a conclusion too soon. Some people are slow to start improving but will get there eventually. You would hate to give up a week too soon, just before your hip was going to start moving more easily with less pain.

Designing Your Own Program

Here are some guidelines to follow for a *safe* progression toward your rehabilitation goals. They are not hard and fast rules—listen to your body. If your pain increases with an exercise, whether that exercise is in the pool or on land, you can move more slowly, perform fewer repetitions, decrease your range of motion (ROM), or skip the exercise altogether. *You* are in charge of your program, which you will design using the pool exercises in chapter 9 and the land exercises in chapter 12. If you've already had hip surgery, turn to chapter 16 and choose from one of two rehab programs: one for recovery from hip arthroscopy and one for hip-implant patients.

Your body's pain messages are the best guide you have while exercising, so listen carefully. But don't expect your body to tell you the same thing every day because your pain's location and severity can change. Begin each day's exercise session slowly, monitoring carefully for possible pain. Make adjustments according to what you feel by moving more slowly or more quickly, reaching for more or less range of motion, and adding or subtracting exercises as appropriate.

You're the one living in that body, working with that challenging hip. It's up to you to discover your own truth about what's possible, what's reasonable, and what's not. Stay alert and keep thinking as you exercise. You will reach some excellent conclusions that will be your own self-created truths.

Guidelines for a Pool and Land Program

Gently try each pool exercise in the order presented. If you don't feel increased hip pain, add that exercise to your program. Skip exercises that increase your pain for now. Try to add them to your program again next week. (You'll be amazed how quickly you gain capability in the water!) Do the low-intensity program of deep-water intervals and the lowest number of repetitions of the other exercises. Increase your intensity and reps gradually each week as long as you don't experience increased hip pain and aren't unduly fatigued. If you're tired or sore on any given day, decrease your intensity and reps.

If you've been exercising four or five times a week in recent months, you can start the first week with three pool *and* two land sessions. These exercises might seem easy compared to a strenuous, abusive exercise regimen, but listen to your body during and after every session. Your hip is the weak link in your body chain right now and needs to be respected. If your hip tells you to back off, ice it right away. If it seems appropriate, you can skip a day of exercising.

Skip pool Exercises 22 to 34 the first month. These jumping exercises could aggravate your hip, so give your body time to gain strength, flexibility, and overall fitness before trying them. When you first do them, wear a flotation belt. After a few weeks, remove the belt and do the jumps gently again. If any of these exercises increases your hip pain, put your belt back on for another week or two.

If you're new to exercising, wait until the second week to add two land sessions to your weekly program. Start with stretching, Exercises 1-6. Then gently try the other exercises in the order presented. If you don't feel increased hip pain, add that exercise to your program. Skip exercises that increase your pain for now. Try to add them to your program again next week. Start with one set of ten reps of each exercise.

Perform only land *or* pool exercises on any given day. You don't want to aggravate your hip by doing too much, so do only one session a day, either pool or land. As you gain strength and capability, you'll add exercises to both your pool and land programs. Soon each of your programs will grow to be quite challenging.

If your hip is sore after a workout, but you "sleep it off" overnight, keep going with your program. However, if you experience pain that does not resolve within twenty-four hours, reconsider. Advanced exercisers should cut their usual program in half until the pain goes away. Beginners can ice the sore hip and wait a day or two before resuming a milder version of the previous exercise sessions.

As your pain decreases and your strength and mobility improve, increase the number of repetitions. In the pool, you can increase your Deep-water Intervals and your Kicking Series by time and the Lower Body Exercises by repetitions. On land, when ten repetitions is no longer challenging, do two sets of ten reps. If you're tired or sore on any given day, decrease your reps.

Most people should allow themselves at least one day of rest during the week. You may be feeling so good that you want to do your exercises every day, but your hip needs time to heal and recover between sessions. If you do the exercises while your muscles are tired or sore you may perform your exercises with improper posture and form, which can lead to further injury to your hip joint and the surrounding tissues. Remember: work + **rest** = improvement. **Plan** the rest days in your program as well as you plan the work days.

If you're used to exercising every day, take one "Active Rest" day the first few weeks. On that day you could take an easy walk, stretch, or do slow pool exercises. You can even do all three as long as you remember it's your recovery day and keep the effort level very low.

Make the mental connection between pool and land. Notice that your body is gaining strength and skill as you run, walk, bend, lift, and squat in the pool. Begin visualizing doing those same movements on land even if you don't yet have enough strength. Soon you'll be doing on land what is so easy in water.

Guidelines for a Land-Only Program

While the ideal is to do the combined pool and land exercise program described, you may not have access to a pool. If you can make the effort to find a pool, you may experience miraculous pain relief starting at your first session. In deep water, your hip will most likely begin moving sooner and with less pain than if you do land exercises **only**. However, if you must have a program you can do at home, here's how to design your land-only program.

Try to begin with three exercise sessions the first week. This is the ideal, but if hip pain has limited your ability to exercise over the past few months, you may need to start with one or two sessions the first week. Listen to your hip as well as the rest of your body. If you're very deconditioned or have trouble doing your normal activities of daily living, do only one to two land exercise sessions a week until the exercises become easy. Then progress to three sessions per week.

Begin with the Exercises 1 to 6. If those stretches feel good to you, do Exercises 7-13. For the first few weeks, perform only one set of ten reps. Let pain be your guide. If an exercise is increasing your pain, decrease your ROM or skip the exercise altogether. If you're performing the exercises properly in your painfree ROM, you should experience very little discomfort doing one set of ten reps.

When you can stand on your affected leg for at least five seconds without pain or instability, you're ready to begin adding the standing exercises, but don't yet add the resistance of a Thera-Band. If you don't feel pain when standing on one leg but balance is a problem, focus on the balance exercises holding a table, counter, or chair until your balance improves.

Thera-Band exercises add resistance to advanced programs. Once you've mastered Exercises 14-17 without resistance, add a Thera-Band to increase your workload. Refer to the chart on page 220 to the progression from easiest color band to the most difficult one.

Refer back to this chapter many times as you learn the pool and land exercises and use them to design your own personalized hip fitness program.

Help for Your Lower Back While Healing Your Hip

When you lose motion and alter your mechanics because of a bad hip, your lower back starts to move abnormally to compensate for what you can no longer do with your hip. That overstresses your back and hurts your disks. But when you get in the water, you begin helping your back as well as any other parts of your body that have suffered. Not only are you working on postponing or avoiding hip surgery, but you are also indirectly helping the other areas that have taken a beating, especially your lower back. One thing we want you to do for sure is avoid back surgery.

—Robert Klapper, MD

Think back to the win-win we discussed as you began your training program and began altering your lifestyle to reduce pain. Despite your best efforts, your pain may be continuing and your mobility may be worsening. If you have done the rehab program for two to three months without major reduction of pain, you may have to conclude that you are no longer going down the Prevention path as you had hoped, but rather are on the Prehab path. Remember, that was the final *win*. You have benefited from increased strength and ability due to your new exercise routines. And now you must refuel your commitment to continue training to be physically powerful enough to withstand the rigors of surgery and recover quickly.

There are two key reasons you may ultimately decide to have hip surgery: First, you're feeling increased symptoms in your hip, such as groin pain waking you from a deep sleep at night. Second, now your back and your knees have started to hurt because you use them to compensate for the lack of motion in your hip. You don't want to ruin joints that are innocent bystanders as you keep trying to save your hip.

At some point, you will begin to build toward the decision for surgery. You and your doctor may realize that the degenerative process has gone too far for any solution other than hip arthroscopy or hip implant surgery, which are explained in chapters 13 and 14.

8

GETTING STARTED IN THE POOL

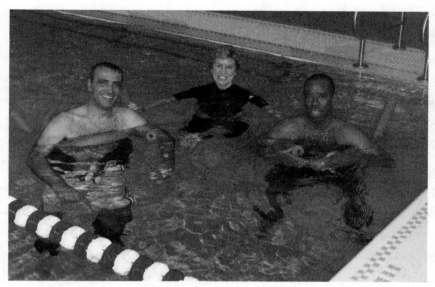

Photo 8-1. Lynda Huey (middle) uses joint distraction with actors
Lorenzo Caccialanza (left) and Courtney B. Vance (right).

When your hip joint becomes disabled, you can't move well, at least not on land; but in water you're able to move in a natural manner. Water's magic lies in its buoyant support for the body, its resistance to bodily movement, the pressure it exerts on a submerged body, its ability to reduce pain, and its relaxing and refreshing feel. As if that isn't enough, it also offers a silent mechanism that we believe is one of its most significant values: by touching your skin, it enhances proprioception, your internal monitoring system of the position of your body parts.

Buoyancy is the upward thrust exerted by water on a body that is totally or partially immersed in it. It lifts the body and provides a feeling of weightlessness. If you stand in waist-deep water, 50 percent of your body weight is supported by the water. If you move to chest-deep water, 70 percent of your body weight is lifted from your weight-bearing joints. In neck-deep water, 90 percent of your body's weight is eliminated, and if you put on a flotation device and move to deep water, you are virtually weightless. By thus neutralizing gravity's downward force on your hips, you are able to exercise in greater comfort and perform movements that are not possible on land.

The resistance the water supplies to the body during movement is considered the workload, just as a stack of weights in the gym is the workload during a weight-training session. Water matches the resistance you give it, which means that the resistance always equals the force you apply. As hard as you push, it pushes back with equal force. This is a safe and efficient way to strengthen even the sorest hip, because you'll never meet more resistance than you can handle.

The amount of resistance the body encounters in water is directly proportional to the speed of the movement. For example, if you move your leg at a slow speed through the water, you feel a gentle resistance. Then if you move your leg exactly twice as fast through the water, you will encounter exactly twice the resistance. The water automatically adapts to your demands and becomes an instantly variable training gym. You can do more or less work, move faster or slower, on any given exercise, depending on what you feel you need.

The hydrostatic pressure exerted by the water on the submerged surfaces of the body is proportional to the depth of submersion. In other words, the deeper you are in the water, the greater the hydrostatic pressure. Think of the water as working on your entire body, like a support stocking works to keep swelling out of your feet, ankles, and calves. Water provides support for unstable joints; it helps venous blood return to the heart, and it relieves swelling, especially in the arms and legs. As you move, the massaging effect of the water on your body helps loosen and lengthen tight muscles while the hydrostatic pressure helps flush out waste products such as lactic acid from tired tissues.

Regaining Motion

Hydrostatic pressure may have another interesting benefit. It may be that the stimulus of the water against your skin enhances the communication between the brain, the nerves, the muscles, and the hip joint. You may have lost some of your sense of position due to injury or arthritis, but it can be enhanced by this different communication link coming from the skin sensors. That new information can help guide you safely through your pool program as you regain motion that has left your movement vocabulary.

The sensation of water on your skin acts as a counterirritant to reduce your pain. Because nerve impulses stimulated by water on your skin are faster than those stimulated by pain, the skin impulses literally beat the pain impulses to the brain for recognition. The end result is reduced pain.

Exercising in water promotes relaxation. The water encourages you to perform gentle, rhythmic motions, which can reduce muscular tension and increase limited range of movement. Further, the mental and emotional stress that comes with pain and impaired physical capability is immediately reduced when you begin movement in water. You perceive less pain and feel more capable, so your body and mind begin to relax.

Benefits of Water Exercise

Exercising in water offers unique benefits to a hip wellness program. You'll feel them as soon as you enter the pool, but first take the time to understand the basic principles at work.

Balanced Strength in Muscle Pairs

Back-and-forth movements of the arms, legs, and trunk are possible only because muscles work in synchronized pairs—when one contracts, the opposing one relaxes. These muscle pairs maintain a specific ratio of strength to each other. If that ratio is thrown out of balance by injury or arthritis, or by training only one of the muscles in a pair, inefficiency and the potential for injury result. Therefore, it is extremely important to exercise both muscles of each antagonistic pair: quadriceps/hamstrings, abductors/adductors, and so forth.

Although you could forget to strengthen one half of a muscle pair on land, that can't happen in the water. Every exercise in water forces you to work both halves of each muscle pair. For every push forward against water's resistance, you must pull backward to the starting position. For every swing upward, you must swing downward. When you exercise in water, symmetry is built in.

Movement Possible Only in Water

In addition to forward and backward and side-to-side movements, the hip joint is capable of a unique circular motion called circumduction. On land there is virtually no way to resist the hip joint evenly as it moves through its complete range of circular movement. In water, however, when your hip performs circumduction, it encounters equal resistance from the water throughout the entire movement, thus gaining maximum strength through its complete range of motion. (See Leg Circles, Exercise 37, page 165.)

Enhanced Proprioception

Proprius in Latin means "one's own," "individual." Perception is awareness. Proprioception means the sense of the relative position of neighboring parts of the body. Your proprioceptors, the Golgi tendon organs, are constantly sending information that is being computed in the brain to provide you with good body awareness. On page 83, you will find a thorough explanation of the unique benefit the water offers as it enhances proprioception.

Aerobic and Anaerobic Fitness

Aerobic fitness allows for moderate, continuous endurance exercise such as hiking for six miles without stopping. Anaerobic fitness is necessary for strenuous bursts of speed and explosive power such as running up a flight of stairs. Both aerobic and anaerobic fitness are vital to a well-conditioned person.

If you suffer from hip pain, it may be impossible for you even to think of performing such activities on land. Continuous aerobic exercise that consists of weight-bearing movements can aggravate your hip through overuse and make your muscles feel heavy. Anaerobic training, by its nature, is powerful, explosive movement that could further damage a deteriorating hip.

In water, however, sore hips are often capable of walking, running, and even jumping so that aerobic work is achieved effortlessly, and anaerobic work sneaks in almost painlessly. You can feel a sense of great strength against the water's resistance, yet because of the greatly reduced gravitational pull, you should be able to finish the workout feeling fresh and having encountered little pain.

Improved Flexibility

Although stretching is a peaceful and soothing activity for most people on land, for some hip patients it produces discomfort and strain. If you avoid most stretches due to hip pain, you will benefit greatly from stretching in water, where comfort and relaxation are built in. You'll find that you can assume positions to perform stretches in the water that you couldn't possibly assume on land. And you can do moving stretches using the water's support and buoyancy that will surprise you with their ease. Further, enjoying stretching means you'll do it more often, for longer periods of time, and with more regularity. That adds up to faster progress.

Increased Range of Motion

The water's buoyancy offers you a somewhat unexpected gift. You'll find that your hip can move forward, backward, and in complete circles much more easily than it ever would be able to on land. This increased range of motion is something you don't have to force. Water's buoyancy will naturally lift your leg higher, wider, and further each session without your having to think about it. This is part of water's magic and what we refer to as the "built-in coach."

Improved Balance

In water you are constantly using your abdominal and back muscles as well as your arms and legs to maintain erect body alignment and balance. Increased strength in these muscles, plus focus on a constantly changing balance point in water, will lead to improved balance on land that will carry over into your daily activities.

Increased Coordination

The brain is complex, with electrical function that is more elegant than a supercomputer. We call the communication between the brain, nerves, and muscles neuromuscular coordination. When you walk or run on land, your right arm and left leg move at the same time: this is called cross-crawl patterning. In water, many people become disoriented regarding the opposition of their limbs. It may take some practice and attention to master this, but the result will be well worth the effort, for water training increases overall coordination by emphasizing cross-crawl patterning, which is the foundation for all human coordination.

Improved Gait

Because of ongoing hip pain, you may have developed an uneven walking pattern or gait, and you may have lost strength in the abductor muscles that stabilize your pelvis. The gait-training exercises starting on page 128 will help you create new habit patterns that are symmetrical and balanced at the same time as they force new strength into the weak muscles.

A Sense of Well-Being

What an amazing change in attitude you can experience as soon as you enter the water! Stress washes away. You'll take a deep breath and notice your shoulders and neck have relaxed. You'll feel better simply for having immersed yourself in water.

The Equipment You'll Need

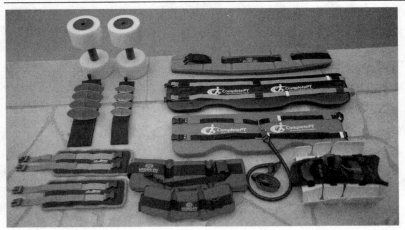

Equipment from top left in clockwise circle: Hydro-Fit Hand Buoys, Hydro-Fit Wave Belt, previous CompletePT Belt, new CompletePT Belt with area for Waterpower Workout Tether Strap to be attached in the midback, Hydro-Tone Boot, Hydro-Fit Buoyancy Cuffs (two sizes), Sprint Ankle Weights, AquaLogix Resistance Blades (two sizes).

See appendix for details.

Your Suit

Men should choose a comfortable pair of trunks. Be sure they have a tie-string to make them snug around the waist so they will stay up when you jump or run. Women should wear one-piece workout suits, not two-piece suits or bikinis. You will be performing a variety of exercises and won't want to be distracted from your form and technique by having to hold your suit in place.

Flotation Belts

Flotation belts support the body in deep water, allowing for full range of motion of both arms and both legs in all body positions, from vertical to horizontal. Every flotation belt has its advantages. Each one has its unique properties that should be considered before making a selection. Choosing the wrong belt can make you uncomfortable in the pool either because it doesn't hold you high enough in the water or because it presses on your rib cage, your chest, or your thighs. If you are under 5'4", you should choose a belt that is narrow at the front: the Wet Sweat Belt, the Wave Belt, or the Aqua Trim Belt. Taller people have more room between their rib cages and hips and therefore can comfortably wear the wider CompletePT Belt. Athletes, dancers, stuntmen, and others who are muscular will need the most possible buoyancy, which is supplied by both the CompletePT and Wet Sweat Belts.

People who are "sinkers"—those with little body fat and dense musculature—need to wear two belts, one on top of the other. While this may feel restrictive and even uncomfortable at first, it's better to be high enough in the water so that you don't lift your chin. As soon as you alter your head position, you affect the entire position of your body. The most comfortable two-belt combination is the CompletePT Belt closest to the body, with the Wave Belt on top, usually turned in the opposite direction to buckle at the back. The CompletePT Belt is best for those with lower back pain because it acts like an orthopedic corset. The Wet Sweat Belt is easiest to pack for travel because it is narrow and dries quickly. (See details of each belt and the table below for a summary of the belts' various features.)

CompletePT Belt. This ensolite foam belt with vinyl coating places buoyancy evenly around the entire waist. The CompletePT Belt is held in place by two narrow canvas straps with quick-release buckles, which allows adjustability in two places for a more comfortable fit. This is the most buoyant of all the belts and should be the belt of choice for use by dancers, athletes, and other "sinkers" who need extra buoyancy. Back patients love the support and sense of security they get from using this belt. They say it feels like wearing a protective corset.

Wet Sweat Belt. A high-buoyancy flotation belt, comfortably narrow at the front with a quick-release buckle. Its narrow construction makes it comfortable during all stretches and exercises. This belt is made of closed-cell foam and covered with vinyl. It dries quickly, making it a good choice for traveling.

Wave Belt. The most comfortable belt due to its narrow construction. A good choice for people under 5'4" or those who don't need extra buoyancy. Also excellent as a second belt for "sinkers" who must wear two in order to keep their chins out of the water during deep-water exercises.

Aqua-Trim Belt. A lightweight, high-buoyancy foam belt with a quick-release buckle. Does the job for those who are watching their budgets.

Flotation Belt Comparison

	Buoyancy Level	Narrow Front	Wide Front	Easy On/Off	Travel Ease
Two-belt combo	highest		✓		hard
CompletePT	high		✓	✓	easy
Wet Sweat	medium	✓		✓	easiest
Aqua-Trim	medium	✓		✓	easy
Wave	low	✓		✓	easy

Support Equipment

When you first learn deep-water exercises, you may have trouble finding your center of balance. A few simple pieces of equipment can make the job of learning these new exercises easier by offering buoyant support.

Hydro-Fit Hand Buoys. One floating Hydro-Fit Hand Buoy in each hand can help you find stability in deep water if that is difficult at first. The buoys allow you to use your upper body strength to help maintain vertical alignment. These Hand Buoys can be held in front of the body, with one on each side of the body, or at any angle in between those two positions.

Hydro-Fit Swim/Therapy Bar. Some people like two small hand buoys while others prefer one long therapy bar to help them maintain their balance in deep water. These tools make it easier to learn new deep-water exercises. The Hydro-Fit Swim/Therapy Bar can also serve as a walker in the pool, providing good support for those doing gait training in chest-deep water.

Buoyancy and Resistance Equipment

Do not use these buoyancy or resistance pieces for the first week of your pool sessions.

Resistance equipment forces you to move more water with each exercise. In effect, this is the equivalent of lifting more weight in the gym and is very effective strength training. Buoyancy cuffs around your ankles help you lift your leg, regaining mobility and motion in your affected hip. If your hip has gone through the Negative Cycle explained on page 22, you will want to add buoyancy pieces to your program by the second week. Use them to regain your normal range of motion. Then, once motion has been restored, you can start using the resistance pieces. If you have relatively normal range of motion in your hip, you can skip the buoyancy and go straight to building strength with the resistance pieces listed below. No resistance equipment should be added to your program until your hip has been pain-free for at least a week.

AquaLogix Resistance Blades. These sturdy, attractive plastic and Velcro pieces strap around the ankles in easy-on, easy-off fashion. They provide three-directional resistance for all hip exercises, meaning that if you want to do leg circles, you have smooth, steady resistance throughout the hip's circumduction. There are two sizes, meaning two levels of resistance. The minimal resistance pieces are called High Speed Blades because athletes can use them against the water's resistance at a much faster pace than the Max Resistance Blades. Don't worry about speed. You may be moving slowly at first, so think of them as the minimal resistance as you work your way up to the maximum resistance equipment.

Hydro-Fit Buoyancy Cuffs. These durable cuffs strap onto the ankles to offer buoyancy during lower body exercises. These are key pieces in helping people regain their full range of motion after hip injury or surgery. The Mini Buoyancy Cuffs get the movement started; the Standard Buoyancy Cuffs challenge the hip further because they offer the equivalent of three to four times the amount of lift.

Hydro-Tone Boots. Using the Hydro-Tone Boots during lower body exercises approximates a weight-training workout. Put your feet into these yellow plastic boots that surround your lower legs and feet and tighten the straps so they fit snugly. The boots interact with the water along all planes of movement. They deliver smooth multidimensional resistance throughout all of the leg movements.

Helpful Equipment

Some additional equipment will add comfort and stability to your pool session. As your pool program becomes a way of life, you may want to invest in these pieces as well.

Pool Shoes. Water shoes can protect your feet and provide traction at the pool, beach, or boat. If you tend to blister easily, or if your pool bottom is slippery, wear pool shoes. If you have diabetes, rheumatoid arthritis, or if you've had hip implant surgery, you should always wear shoes, not only in the pool but going to and from the pool as well. You want to take every precaution not to step on anything and get an infection. You can find these online or during the summer months at your local drug or sporting goods store.

Waterpower Workout Tether and Strap. This well-constructed tether has a sturdy nylon waistband that is attached to a length of canvas and latex tubing. It fits snugly over your flotation device and attaches from your waist to the side of the pool. If you're having trouble establishing good deep-water running and walking form, the tether will offer you stability and significantly improve your posture. In shallow water, the tether lets you run at top speed without slipping or moving around the pool.

You might worry, especially after hip surgery, that a stray swimmer won't notice you and bump into you. You can make your location known to all swimmers by tethering yourself in one spot and staying there while you do your deep-water exercises. If you choose the CompletePT Belt, the Aqua Trim Belt, or the Wave Belt, you can buy just the Waterpower Workout Strap. Hook the tether strap directly onto the belt strap and eliminate the need for the waistband when doing Deep-Water Intervals. The waistband and the strap are both needed for shallow water running.

Clothing to Keep You Warm

When you first begin the hip pool program, you may be moving quite slowly. If your pool temperature is the standard 82 to 84 degrees, you'll probably find yourself getting cold and starting to shiver within twenty minutes. In order to be comfortable in cool water, consider investing in a surfer-like piece of attire that is specifically designed to keep you warm. Pullover Thermo X Shirts are fleece-lined, stretch, and offer protection from the sun's UV rays as well as a luxurious layer of warmth against cool water. They come in either long-sleeved or short-sleeved styles. A Neoprene, short-sleeve, zip-up shirt is even warmer. The Hydro-Fit Shirt is stylish as it protects against UV rays and offers a thin layer of warmth against the cold. Use the Thermo Shirt if you're feeling slightly chilled, but put on a shorty wet suit if you're downright cold. (All attire is listed in the appendix except wet suits. You can buy them online or find them in surf shops and dive shops.)

The Pool

You may have one in your backyard or at your gym. You may have to search to find one that will provide you with the depth of water you need and the appropriate temperature. This search is a worthy effort, for pool therapy may save you thousands of dollars in other kinds of treatments. While you look, keep an eye open for pools with deep water where you can take all your weight off your sore hip. Although you can exercise in chest-deep water, you aren't as likely to experience the immediate and miraculous sensation of pain reduction from your first pool session as when you are in deep water.

Nearly every community has a pool that can be used for a small fee. Your local college, YMCA, YWCA, Jewish Community Center, and recreation department are your best bets for finding inexpensive access to pools. Health club membership fees can be expensive, but they usually include plush facilities such as a sauna, steam room, or Jacuzzi. Hotels may offer pool memberships to the neighborhood.

The pool you use for hip rehabilitation should have a shallow end with chest-deep water for your specific height. For example, if you are five feet three inches, chest-deep water is approximately three feet nine inches. If you are six feet tall, chest-deep water is closer to four feet six inches. You ideally want to have a relatively flat or unslanted pool bottom so you can walk across the pool at that correct depth. Besides chest-deep water, you'll also need water that is so deep your feet won't touch the bottom of the pool. For most people, this means you need water at least six feet deep.

CompletePT's Ideal Pool

We designed our 92-degree, saltwater pool in West Los Angeles with ideal shallow and deep ends. Half the pool is deep and half the pool is shallow. We have a unique double-bar system on both sides of the pool for tethering, stretching, and kicking. Our non-swimmers hold on to the bars, feeling secure as they venture into deep water with both hands on the top bar. Students in our group classes and our physical therapy patients have the optimum amenities for water exercise and therapy.

—Lynda Huey

When you first begin your program, you might be moving quite slowly. Water temperatures of 88 to 90 degrees will be most comfortable for you. As you progress and begin moving more strenuously, you'll feel comfortable in water that is 84 to 87 degrees in temperature. Unfortunately, most people don't have access to the perfect pool or control of the ideal water temperature, so if you have to decide between the two, choose a pool that has the proper depth of water for you even if the water is cooler than you'd like. You can always make yourself warmer with additional protective clothing as mentioned above.

Check your potential pool's schedule. Make sure there is a recreational swim time during which you can use the pool without interference from lap-swimmers, children, or divers. Ideally, the pool you choose for your water training should be no more than ten to fifteen minutes from your home or workplace. The locker room should be clean, inviting, and comfortable. If your "home" pool is easily accessible, and if you are comfortable in its surroundings, you'll go more often than if it's unattractive or a long drive away. Next, find a backup pool for emergency use. You'd hate to find an unexpected Closed sign on your main pool and have to miss your aquatic therapy for a week or two just because you hadn't located an alternate pool.

If You Build Your Own Pool

Many people eventually decide to build their own backyard pools to meet their specific needs. If you make the decision to build your own pool, consider these ideas in your planning:

- Think of the annual weather pattern in your area. If you don't have at least four to five months of weather good enough for outdoor pool exercise, think again. A small indoor tank or health club membership might be more appropriate for you.
- Consider the amount of sunlight you have in your backyard. You don't want a pool that's in the shade all day, but rather one that's mostly in the sun.
- Pay attention to the surrounding trees and think of how much wind you have coming from which prevailing direction. Consider the leaves, flowers, or other droppings that will fall into your pool, depending on where you place it.
- Ask friends and business associates for names of reputable pool builders. Interview at least three builders and get names of pool owners in your area whom you can visit to see their pools and ask questions about the building process.

- Plan approximately equal amounts of shallow and deep water in your pool. Without the appropriate depth of shallow water, you can't do the Gait Training, Impact Exercises, or Lower Body Exercises well. Without deep water, you're not able to do non-weight-bearing exercises.
  - If your pool will be relatively small, you may need to ask the builder to create a flat, non-slanted shallow end so that you can do your gait training in chest-deep water. Measure from the ground to the middle of your chest to see exactly how deep your shallow water should be. If two or more people of differing heights intend to use the pool, you may have to compromise by selecting an average chest-height depth.
  - The deep end should have water deep enough so that your feet won't touch the bottom of the pool. For most people, this means you need water at least six feet deep. When building small pools, you may have to ask your city for a variance to the standard pool-building permit so that you can have one unvarying depth in the shallow end, then let the bottom make a 90-degree drop off into the deep end.
- Place therapy bars on the walls in both the deep and shallow ends to hold during stretching and kicking exercises. Face them away from the dominant direction of the sun.
- Plan your stairs into the pool to have a shorter rise than normal stairs. For instance, make four easy steps down into the pool rather than three steeper steps.
- Add two railings going down your stairs so you can walk between them. You can hold one bar in each hand and comfortably lower yourself down the steps. If you build a spa, add another set of railings to help you in and out.
- Design a square or rectangular pool so an electric cover can easily be installed to keep your pool warm a few extra months each year or even year-round. Odd-shaped pools can make adding a pool cover virtually impossible. If you add a spa, place it inside the pool perimeter so it, too, can be covered when not in use.
- Consider solar heating, which in the long run will cut down your gas bill for heating the water.

Guidelines for the Pool Program

Before you begin the pool program in chapter 9, give some consideration to the physical limitations imposed by your hip. You'll want to be mindful of its condition each time you're in the pool and adjust your session accordingly. You'll also want to make notes of aches or pains you feel with specific movements, then observe the increase in your capabilities as your pain reduces over the next weeks and months.

- **If you have had hip surgery, turn to chapter 10.** That is where you will find your post-surgical exercises. Chapter 16 offers you a protocol with pool and land exercises as you recover from hip arthroscopy or hip implant surgery. Skip chapter 9. You'll appreciate the encouragement and cautions supplied in chapters 10 and 16.
- **Let your body tell you which exercises you can do.** Your body's pain messages are the best guide you have while exercising. Listen carefully. Don't expect your body to tell you the same thing every day because the location and severity of your pain can change.
- **If you feel a sharp pain, stop what you're doing immediately.** Try making the same movement at a much slower pace. If that doesn't eliminate the pain, narrow the range of motion of that exercise. If moving more slowly or working through a narrower range of motion doesn't bring your pain level down significantly, don't do that particular exercise today. Try it again slowly next week.
- **Respect the weakest link in your body "chain."** Your hip is the weak link at the moment. Any exercise you do should move at the pace tolerated by that hip.
- **Underdo anything new.** Begin slowly, monitoring carefully for possible pain. Because you feel less pain in the water, and because you may not feel the pain of a new movement until the next day, perform fewer repetitions than you think you can tolerate and at a slower pace.
- **Do it first in the water.** Whatever you may be planning to do on land, try it out first in the pool, where you'll be less likely to hurt your hip. Try a golf or tennis swing; try bending and reaching as you would at work. Remind your body what you expect of it before adding gravity.

Correct Biomechanics

Whether you sit, stand, walk, run, or perform any other activity, there is a position, posture, stance, or alignment that helps the body perform the activity most smoothly and with the least effort or strain. If you use correct biomechanics, or good form, your movements will be more efficient. When you first begin your pool program, focus on good form before adding speed. Here are some general rules of good biomechanics:

- **Never work faster than good form will allow.** If your form crumbles during any of the exercises, particularly the deep-water running and walking, slow down and put the building blocks together again from the beginning.
- **Find a focal point at eye level**. By keeping your eyes focused on that point, your head will be less likely to bob or weave. Holding your head steady helps you keep your shoulders and hips steady. If your chin tilts up, your back automatically arches and your hips sway back. If your chin tilts down, your body tends to curl up.
- **Try to isolate the muscles involved in each exercise.** Don't move other body parts to generate a "whipping" action for added strength. For example, when doing leg circles, many people swing their entire bodies in order to move the leg. Instead, hold the rest of your body stable while you use only the muscles surrounding the hip to do the work. That way you'll gain more strength exactly where you targeted it.

Tips for Improving Your Pool Sessions

- Establish your space in the pool.
- Ignore curious onlookers.
- Keep your goals firmly in mind.
- Concentrate on your movements.
- Have fun in the water.

9

A POOL PROGRAM FOR HIP PATIENTS

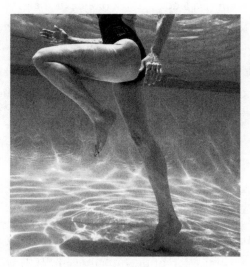

Photo 9-2. Marching.

You can gain wonderful, perhaps unexpected benefits from exercising your affected hip. If you are willing to commit to the following aquatic therapy program, your entire body will eventually be in great shape. You will become stronger and more flexible, have better cardiovascular capacity, move more efficiently, and will simply feel better. *If you've had hip surgery in the past six months, start with chapter 10, where you will find the necessary concepts, encouragements, and cautions to guide you.*

This program can be the reason you never have a hip surgery. The exercises included here can help you turn that concept into a reality. Or you may suspect surgery is on your horizon in the long run, but you're hoping to prevent it for the short run. Good for you for thinking ahead and learning the exercises in advance! Not only will you reduce your pain and improve the function of your hip, but you will improve your overall fitness in preparation for surgery. And you will master these exercises before you would have to try them with post-surgical concerns. These exercises will become your usual routine. By learning them now, you won't be nervous at all when it's time to climb into the pool after surgery.

We have learned over the years that almost miraculous benefits can come from doing deep-water exercises. But not everyone is willing to be in deep water. This program contains exercises in both deep and shallow water. If you're a non-swimmer or afraid of the water, start with the Gait Training Exercises 1 through 3. You'll start in shallow water and won't need a flotation belt. Over time you will gain confidence in the water and may be able to add deep-water exercises to your program. Many non-swimmers do because they feel secure holding on to a ladder, gutter, or side of the pool. In our pool, where therapists are side by side in the water with the patients, *all* of our patients move to the deep water, where they hold on to our therapy bars. We understand the incredible benefits of taking all the weight off a sore hip, so we coax even the most fearful patient to experience that. Once they do, they receive benefits that far outweigh their fear, and thereafter find it easier to summon up their courage to keep moving to deep water. There are two deep-water sections in this program. We'll advise you along the way if you wish to skip them for now.

Gait Training

You may have damaged your hip in a sudden injury, or it may have taken months or years for your hip condition to develop. Either way, you have probably found that your normal walking pattern has become irregular due to pain or limitation of the hip's movement. If walking on land causes you hip pain or discomfort, you'll find it a welcome relief to have most of your weight lifted off your hip joint while you walk in the water. In chest-deep water, you can walk relatively pain-free and at the same time relearn or refine the correct biomechanics of walking.

If your pool bottom is slippery or if your feet tend to blister easily, wear pool shoes to provide traction and protection. If you have diabetes, rheumatoid arthritis, or have had a hip implant operation, always wear pool shoes to prevent a cut that could become infected.

Walk back and forth across the width of a pool, if possible, so that you will have the same depth of water and the same amount of water resistance throughout the exercise. You can still get the job done if you must walk the length of the pool in one lane, but you will find yourself constantly adjusting to a changing amount of buoyancy and resistance due to the changing depth of the water.

Before performing Exercises 1 through 3, spend a moment trying to visualize yourself walking tall, straight, and without any limp or deviation in your gait. Picture your feet and knees always facing forward and your hips and shoulders always level, never bobbing up and down or rocking from side to side. Then begin with Exercise 1. Perform each of the walking exercises for three or four pool crossings during the first few sessions. This is your warm-up while your body adapts to the water temperature.

Exercise 1. Shallow-Water Walking—Forward, Backward, Sideways

Face the center of the pool and prepare to take your first small steps forward onto the sore hip. If you feel pain in the affected hip when you step on it, try the basic modifications shown in the box above. Take one small step, then another, moving your arms and legs in time with each other. Try to move your right arm at the same time as your left leg and move your left arm with your right leg. If this cross-crawl pattern (see page 115) is too difficult to master right now, let your arms float comfortably at your sides for balance. Eventually you do want to learn to walk with opposition between your arms and legs, but that isn't your first priority—walking without a limp is. Cross the pool several times walking with small steps until all gait irregularities are gone. Then you can begin lengthening your steps. After crossing the pool several times, try walking backward.

Face the side of the pool. Look to see that you have an unobstructed space behind you, then begin walking backward. Don't worry about your arms while walking backward. If you feel pain when you step on the affected hip, try the basic modifications. Walk slowly across the pool, turn, and continue walking backward across the pool again. Keep your steps short until you can walk without a limp, then gradually lengthen them.

Next, walk sideways across the pool, starting by pushing off with your unaffected leg and stepping onto the affected leg. Bring the unaffected leg to a closed position. Step and close, step and close in this manner across the pool, starting with small steps. Look down at your feet. Many people incorrectly turn their feet in the direction they are stepping. Constantly check your feet to make sure they are parallel to each other and pointing straight forward. If you encounter any pain, move to deeper water, take smaller steps, or put on your flotation belt. Don't lurch or lean from side to side. Rather, keep your shoulders and hips level throughout the sideways walking. When you've crossed the pool, *keep facing in the same direction*, so that as you re-cross the pool, you will push off with the opposite leg.

Exercise 2. Marching

You don't need to lift your knee as high as in Photo 9-2. This is a goal to strive for, but it may not be where you begin.

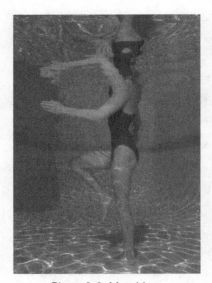

Photo 9-2. Marching.

Begin marching by lifting one of your knees as high as you can without hip discomfort or pain. If you encounter pain, that's the "red line" mentioned in the box above. Lean forward and take a step, then lift the other knee to a similar position.

If you feel pain in the affected hip and you've tried the basic modifications in the box on page 189, don't lift your knee so high. Pay attention to the direction your knees are pointing while you march. Perhaps your right knee is pointing straight forward while your left knee points slightly to the left side or across the midline of your body. Try to correct the movement so that both knees point straight forward. If the full correction causes increased hip pain, adjust the correction back to the point of no pain, thus returning to a position that is comfortable. You can aim toward better alignment again next time. Use bent arms in opposition to the bent knees. Your right arm should move in time with your left knee, and your left arm should move with your right knee.

Exercise 3. Long-Leg Walk

This exercise may be too difficult for you at first if your hip has lost much function. You can wait a few weeks before adding it to your program.

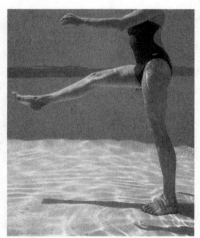

Walking forward, lift your straight right leg toward the surface of the water and reach your left arm forward for balance and opposition. (See Photo 9-3.) Continue this long-leg walk across the pool, swinging your arms forcefully through the water in opposition to your legs. Don't worry if you can't lift your leg as high as in the photo. Keep your leg straight and lift it as high as you comfortably can.

Photo 9-3. Long-Leg Walk.

If you do not yet have a flotation belt, or if you wish to skip the deep-water exercises, move to the Stretching section on page 139.

Deep-Water Intervals

Most people will need a few sessions to learn the balance and rhythm of each of these exercises since they are unfamiliar movements. Learn Deep-Water Running, Power Walk, and Flies (Exercises 4 through 6). If you become stable with those three, then you can add Speed Walk (Exercise 7). *Lynda Huey's Waterpower Workout* video offers underwater footage to help you learn the exercises. Those who want to focus on their interval training should consider adding a tether as shown in these photos, which helps improve good form. The video and all the equipment in this chapter are listed in the appendix at the back of the book.

Do the medium-intensity program the first session. If it seems too difficult, move to low intensity right away. If the medium intensity seems too easy, don't move up to the high-intensity program until the next session. You won't know until the next day whether your hip or your muscles are going to be sore or whether you will become overly fatigued.

Exercise 4. Deep-Water Running

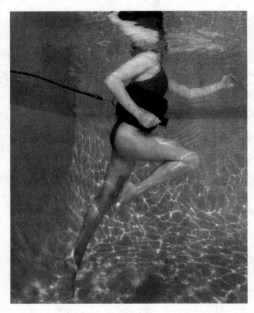

Photo 9-4A.
Deep-Water Running using a tether.

Run in an upright position using the same arm motion of good running form on land. Your legs do only the back half of the running motion. Lift each knee, then push each foot straight down behind you as in Photo 9-4A. Focus your eyes on a point straight ahead that will help you keep your head level and unmoving. Keep your chest erect and your shoulders relaxed and down. Lift each knee so that your thigh is at a 90-degree angle to your body, or as high as your hip will allow if 90 degrees causes you pain. Pull your arms forward and backward with no lateral movement. Relax your hands, palms facing inward, not down, and pull your elbows straight back, each in its turn. Don't lean too far forward or you'll be dog paddling.

Can't swim? If you're a non-swimmer or if this seems too challenging a way to begin, you can hold on to the side of the pool. Perhaps the best place to hold is in the corner so that when you lift your knee, you don't have to worry about hitting the pool wall. See Photo 9-4B.

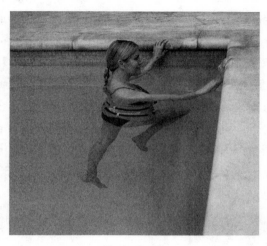

Photo 9-4B.
Deep-Water Running holding the corner of the pool.

You can also try a marching or bicycling motion if the running proves difficult. For marching, you lift your knees straight up and push your feet straight down within a range of motion that does not cause discomfort. For bicycling, you can start with a small cycling motion, then increase the size of your cycle as you regain mobility. Bicycling is the easiest, so if you started there, move to marching in a few weeks if you can, then eventually work your way into running.

Start Deep-Water Walking Slowly

A lot of force is required to swing straight legs through the water's resistance as in Exercise 5, which comes next. It is possible to strain your hip flexor muscles from working too fast too soon, so begin slowly and increase your speed very gradually over several weeks.

—Lynda Huey

Exercise 5. Deep-Water Walking—Basic Walk and Power Walk

Start in an upright position with no forward or backward lean. Hold your right arm and your left leg forward at the same time to establish your "opposition" position as in Photo 9-5A. Then begin an exaggerated walking motion, one in which the knees never bend. Swing your arms and legs forward and backward—right arm with left leg and left arm with right leg—in a smooth, flowing motion. This is the Basic Walk.

For Power Walk, turn your hands so the palms face backward and are wide like paddles. This creates increased resistance for your shoulders, chest, and back. In order to create more work for your calf muscles, flex the foot on the leg that swings forward and point the foot on the leg that swings backward. One foot is flexing and one is pointing on each step as in Photo 9-5B.

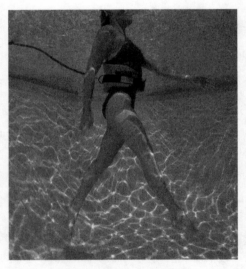

Photo 9-5A. Deep-water Basic Walk.

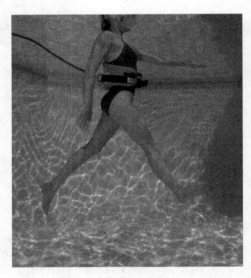

Photo 9-5B. Power Walk.

Exercise 6. Flies

Assume the position shown in Photo 9-6A with your hands and feet together. Your feet are relaxed and your palms face down just beneath the surface of the water. Slice your hands through the water as you reach your arms to the side. At the

HEAL YOUR HIPS

same time, open your legs to the position in Photo 9-6B. Return with equal force to the starting position. Don't push your hands deeper into the water. You want minimal resistance on your hands and arms to prevent bobbing up and down.

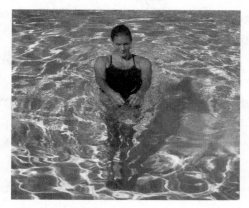

Photo 9-6A. Flies.

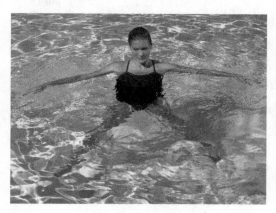

Photo 9-6B.

If you've noticed limited motion in one or both hips, you may want to try adding ankle weights to each leg as you do this exercise. You can hold on to the side of the pool at first if you wish. This slight joint distraction to the hip can surprise you: you may experience less pain and greater range of motion.

Notice in Photos 9-6C and 9-6D that an extra flotation belt has been added to counteract the downward pull of the weights. Once you master this basic exercise with ankle weights, try to perform external and internal hip rotations by turning your toes out as you open your legs, and turning your toes in as you bring your legs back together. To remember how to do this, say to yourself, "Toes out on the way out. Toes in on the way in."

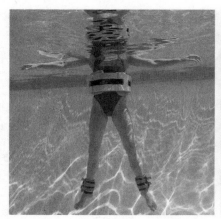

Photo 9-6C. External Rotation.

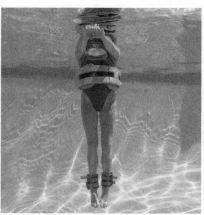

Photo 9-6D. Internal Rotation.

A POOL PROGRAM FOR HIP PATIENTS

Exercise 7. Speed Walk

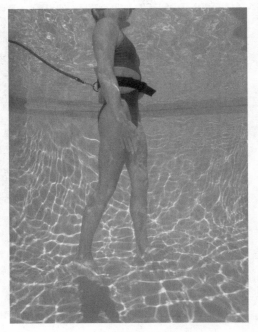

Photo 9-7. Speed Walk.

Turn your hands with the thumbs forward so that your hands "slice" through the water. Your elbows and knees remain straight throughout the exercise. Tighten your abdominal muscles and your **gluteal** muscles to create a solid torso from which to rapidly swing your arms and legs. Lift your toes so that your feet are flat as if you were standing on land. This will help you keep your knees straight. Narrow the forward and backward range of motion of your legs so they swing forward and backward less than a foot or so as in Photo 9-7. Now quicken your steps as you firmly hold your opposition position. If your shoulders begin to wobble, you've lost the opposition. Slow down and start again, gradually building the speed.

Exercise 8. Deep-Water Intervals

You will use the skills you learned in Exercises 4 through 7 to create a powerful cardiovascular series. At the same time you'll be developing good biomechanics while you strengthen all the muscles that surround your hips.

Interval training involves performing a challenging work period, then resting, then working again. Running and Walking are used as the work periods, while Flies are used as the recovery periods. At first you may not be challenging your cardiovascular system and may not require much of a rest period. However, as your hip heals and can withstand more force, you'll be able to increase the effort and speed of these intervals and raise your working heart rate to whatever level you desire.

All these intervals start with low intensity and move to higher intensity. If you feel an increase in pain in your hip at any time, slow down. If you have any concerns for your heart, discuss this program with your physician before beginning and monitor your heart rate when suggested.

Measuring Your Heart Rate

To measure your heart rate, count the number of beats you feel at your carotid artery in your neck for six seconds. Add a zero to find your heart rate. Not only is this the easiest way to compute your heart rate, but recent studies have shown it to be more accurate than counting for ten seconds and multiplying by six.

Low-Intensity Program

Water Run (slow), one minute

Basic Walk or Power Walk (slow), one minute

Flies, thirty seconds

Water Run (slow), two minutes

Basic Walk or Power Walk (slow), two minutes

(Heart-rate check)

Flies, thirty seconds

Repeat this sequence once or twice per your tolerance.

Total time: seven minutes, once; fourteen minutes (if repeated)

Medium-Intensity Program

Water Run (slow), one minute

Water Run (moderate), one minute

Flies, thirty seconds

Water Run (slow), one minute

Water Run (moderate), one minute

Basic Walk or Power Walk (moderate), one minute

(Heart-rate check)

Flies, thirty seconds

Basic Walk or Power Walk (slow), one minute

Basic Walk or Power Walk (moderate), one minute

Water Run (moderate), one minute

(Heart-rate check)

Flies, thirty seconds

Power Walk (slow), thirty seconds

Speed Walk (fast), thirty seconds

Flies, thirty seconds

(Heart-rate check)

Repeat this sequence if your stamina and your hip allow.

Total time: eleven minutes or twenty-two minutes (if repeated)

High-Intensity Program

Even if your fitness level can handle a high-intensity series of intervals, you must remember to defer to your hip. If working fast and hard against the water resistance increases the pain in your hip, *slow down*. If running is easier on your hip than walking, do your fastest, hardest intervals in running mode and your slower and more moderate intervals while walking. Skip Speed Walk altogether if it causes too much pain. Over the weeks, try gradually to reintroduce Speed Walk to your program.

Water Run, one-minute buildup, increasing pace every fifteen seconds to create a four-speed
  interval: slow, medium, fast, sprint

(Heart-rate check)

Flies, thirty seconds

Repeat Water Run, one-minute buildup: slow, medium, fast, sprint

(Heart-rate check)

Flies, thirty seconds

Power Walk (moderate), one minute

Power Walk (hard), thirty seconds

(Heart-rate check)

Flies, thirty seconds

Power Walk (moderate), one minute

Speed Walk (fast), thirty seconds

(Heart-rate check)

Flies, thirty seconds

Run (fast), thirty seconds

Power Walk (hard), thirty seconds

Speed Walk (fast), thirty seconds

(Heart-rate check)

Flies, thirty seconds

Water Run (fast), one minute

Power Walk (hard), one minute

Speed Walk (fast), thirty seconds

(Heart-rate check)

Flies, thirty seconds

Repeat this sequence if your stamina and your hip allow.

Total time: twelve minutes or twenty-four minutes (if repeated)

Gradually increase the difficulty of your interval session over the next weeks and months. Use what you've learned about interval training from the examples above to create your own personalized interval session that lasts fifteen to thirty minutes. Vary your session from day to day to avoid losing interest.

Stretching

Stretching reduces muscle tension and makes your body feel more relaxed. It increases the range of motion of your hip joint while it helps you get to know your own body better: As you stretch, you receive messages from your body. Listen to these messages carefully.

Never force a stretch if there is pain. Stretch only to the point of discomfort to find your limit. Then ease back a bit and hold a challenging stretching position while you breathe slowly and deeply to assist the stretching process.

Turn to face the side of the pool for Stretching Exercises 9 through 13. If you perform them in deep water, wear a flotation device. If you do them in shallow water, you won't need one.

Is One Side More Flexible?

Don't be surprised to find that one leg or one side of your body is more flexible than the other. You can address that imbalance by spending more time stretching the tight side. The easiest way to do that is to stretch the tight side first, then the other side, then return to the tight side for a final stretch.

—Lynda Huey

Exercise 9. Hamstring Stretch

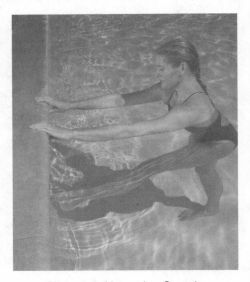

Photo 9-9. Hamstring Stretch.

Grasp the side of the pool with both hands as shown in Photo 9-9. Start with your unaffected hip. Place your foot, toes up, against the pool wall. Keep your neck, shoulders, arms, and back relaxed throughout the exercise. Gently straighten your knee as far as you can while you breathe deeply and slowly five times. Now try this more carefully stretching the affected side. You may need to lower your foot on the pool wall to remain pain-free. Over the next weeks and months, try to push your heel toward the pool wall with the goal of making contact.

Exercise 10. Body Swing

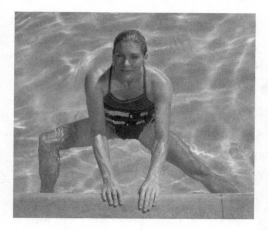

Photo 9-10. Body Swing.

Continue grasping the side of the pool. Bend both knees and walk your feet partway up the pool wall. Place your feet comfortably apart with your knees just outside your elbows. Stay on the balls of your feet with your toes slightly turned out. If you keep both heels flat on the wall, you won't be able to do this exercise. Keeping your hands and feet in the same place, bend your right knee and let your body swing to the right as in Photo 9-10. Your left heel will go flat against the wall, and your right heel will lift farther away from the wall.

Now straighten your right knee, push yourself to the left, and bend your left knee. Your left heel will lift off, and your right heel will go flat to the wall. Slowly continue swinging back and forth, paying attention to what you feel as you swing right and left. Each right-left swing is one repetition. Do four to six repetitions, working on gaining more movement in your problematic hip. If you feel the need to stop and push into the stretch on your sore hip, do it slowly while breathing deeply.

Exercise 11. Lateral Split

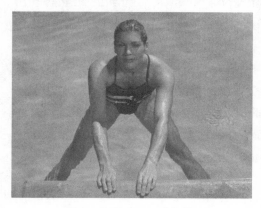

Photo 9-11. Lateral Split.

Continue grasping the side of the pool. Gradually walk your feet away from each other, opening your legs to the side as far as you comfortably can as in Photo 9-11. If the position is too comfortable, stretch slightly farther. If the position is painfully uncomfortable, move your feet closer together. Hold this position while you take five slow, deep breaths. As you improve at this stretch, you can make it more difficult by leaning your upper body forward toward the pool wall.

Exercise 12. Quad Stretch

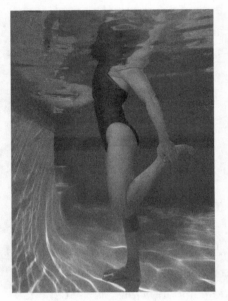

Photo 9-12. Quad stretch.

Hold the side of the pool for balance with your right hand. Grasp your left ankle with your left hand and slowly pull the left heel toward the buttocks as shown in Photo 9-12. Keep the knees close together, and make sure you haven't gone into a sway-back position. Breathe deeply five times as you feel the muscles relax and lengthen. Switch sides. Hold on to the side of the pool with your left hand and repeat with the right leg.

Exercise 13. Hip Flexor Stretch

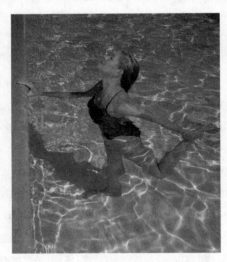

Photo 9-13. Hip Flexor Stretch.

Start in the same position as for Exercise 12. Keep your left elbow straight as you allow your left knee to swing straight backward to the position shown in Photo 9-13. Lift up through the rib cage to increase the stretch. If you have a lower back problem, this is where you will remain. Otherwise, look up at the ceiling for an even deeper stretch of the hip flexors. Breathe slowly and deeply five times, then repeat on the other side.

HEAL YOUR HIPS

If you do not yet have a flotation belt, or if you wish to skip the deep-water exercises, move to the Kicking Series section on page 104.

Deep-Water Exercises

If these exercises are hard for you to do as shown, or if you're a non-swimmer, you can hold on to the side of the pool. Start all exercises slowly. Then, if you feel no hip pain, gradually increase your effort level. Start with ten repetitions of each. If that feels easy, do fifteen or twenty reps the next time. If performed consistently, these three exercises can help you regain freedom of motion in your hip. But don't push into an area of pain. Stop just as you start to feel discomfort, then back away. Over the weeks, you can expect to start moving farther with more effort and less discomfort.

Exercise 14. Bent-Knee Twists

If you are following hip implant precautions, skip this exercise and follow the protocol that begins on page 306.

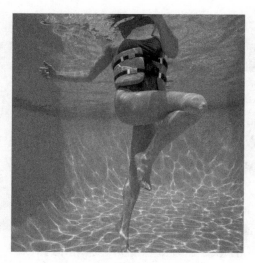

Slightly bend both arms at the elbows. Lift your right knee across your body toward your left elbow, then your left knee toward your right elbow. They probably won't touch, but you want to have your upper body twisting one way and your lower body twisting the opposite way. Each right-left sequence counts as one repetition.

Photo 9-14. Bent-Knee Twists.

Exercise 15. Straight-Leg Twists

If you are following hip implant precautions, skip this exercise and follow the protocol that begins on page 306.

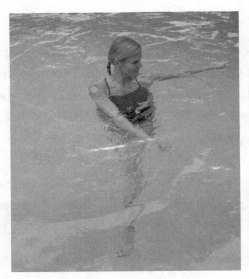

Photo 9-15. Straight-Leg Twists.

Straighten your arms and legs, and continue the twisting movement as in Exercise 14. This time, reach not just toward the left leg but well past it as in Photo 9-15. Continue by reaching your left hand well past your right leg. You may need to lean slightly backward and lift your legs a bit in order to achieve the correct balance for this exercise. The farther you reach on each twist, the more completely you will stretch your hips and strengthen the muscles around them. Keep both legs completely straight throughout the entire exercise.

Exercise 16. V-Kicks

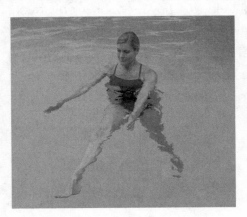

Photo 9-16. V-Kicks.

This exercise can be tricky to learn, so here's the easiest progression. Start by doing a Basic Walk as in Exercise 5. Next, lean back slightly and lift your legs halfway to the surface as you keep walking. Then open your legs slightly apart to create the V as you swing both arms toward the leg that lifts as in Photo 9-16. Keep both legs straight throughout the entire exercise. You can make this exercise easier or harder by altering your hand and arm positions. If your elbows are bent, and your hands are relaxed, that will be the easiest version with the least resistance. As you move your hands farther away from your body to the straight position shown in the photo, that will be harder. Tighten your abdominals and other muscles of your torso because you'll need to maintain strong core stabilization the harder you swing your arms. Finally, if you turn your hands so your thumbs face up toward the ceiling and you hold your hands firm like paddles, you will have reached the variation for maximum resistance.

Kicking Series

Speed Kicks and Power Kicks

In the past few years, I have begun thinking of the kicking series in two categories: Speed Kicks and Power Kicks. The Speed Kicks for hips are Exercise 17, Back Flutter, and Exercise 18, Bicycling. The Power Kicks for hips are Exercise 19, Deep Back Kicks; Exercise 20, Straight-Leg Deep Kick; and Exercise 21, Scissors. The Speed Kicks are just what they sound like—you do them *fast*. Or at least you work your way up to top speed over weeks and months. The Power Kicks are larger, more forceful movements, so you can add resistance pieces to your ankles while doing them, which forces the muscles to work harder. It's the equivalent of increasing the weights you lift in the weight room. Never use resistance pieces in the first few sessions. Work into them. When the Power Kicks start feeling easy, that's the time to add the Aqualogix Blades or Hydro-Tone Boots. (See appendix for details.)

—Lynda Huey

You can do Exercises 17 through 21 either in deep water or shallow. You can hold on to the sides of the pool, lean your back into a corner, or sit on a step. If you brace yourself on the side of the pool, experiment to find the most comfortable position for your shoulders. That position may change from exercise to exercise. You will most likely perform the kicks better if you are wearing a flotation belt. These kicks target the hips, thighs, buttocks, and core muscles for strengthening. If you feel hip pain, slow your kicking movements or narrow your range of motion. If you still feel pain, stop the exercise you are doing but gently try the next one. Retry the kick that caused pain next week. You'll soon be able to do it.

Exercises 19 and 20 are best performed in deep water. If you do them in shallow water, you'll have to modify your movements so you lightly tap your feet on the pool bottom, but then immediately return to the essence of the kick as shown.

Speed Kicks

Do each of these kicks for one minute. If you don't have a clock with a second hand by your pool, consider buying a cheap one and setting it up on a plastic stand on the deck. Being able to see how much more time you have to work on each kick will help you pace yourself at the proper effort level. If you don't have a second hand to watch, do thirty to fifty repetitions of each.

Once you've learned the Speed Kicks and want to take them up a notch, move to an unused corner of the pool where your splashing won't disturb others. Try to time it right so that you have about twenty feet of empty pool in all directions when you do your speed kicks. It might mean coming to the pool early or staying late. Do whatever it takes to have *this much fun*! These kicks have been the favorite of some of the world's best athletes. You will find out why.

Exercise 17. Back Flutter Kicks

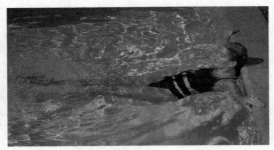

Photo 9-17. Back Flutter Kicks.

Brace yourself with your back to the pool wall and your arms on the gutter or edge of the pool. Lay your head back on the deck as in Photo 9-17. Lift your hips and legs, and begin shallow flutter kicks with straight legs. On days when your hip is sore, keep your feet under the water for less stress on the joint. Otherwise, when you're doing this comfortably, start breaking the surface of the water with your feet to create more workload. Keep your ankles relaxed so your feet move up and down on each kick. Kick for one minute or do fifty right-left repetitions.

Athletes: Kick hard for the first thirty seconds, then kick at maximum effort level for the last thirty seconds.

HEAL YOUR HIPS

Continue bracing yourself at the side of the pool, or go to a corner or step as in Photos 9-18A and 9-18B. Bend your knees to begin kicking in a bicycling movement. You may need to close your eyes during this one since it creates the most white water. Do forty right-left repetitions.

Athletes: *Start this one slowly so you don't get a hamstring cramp!* World-class sprinters and jumpers will often cramp if they start at their fastest pace without building up slowly. Build up your speed for the first thirty seconds, then lift your feet out of the water to increase the size of the cycling motion. As your speed escalates, pull your heels quickly toward your buttocks on each cycle.

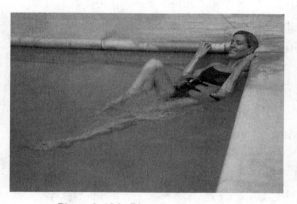

Photo 9-18A. Bicycling in a corner.

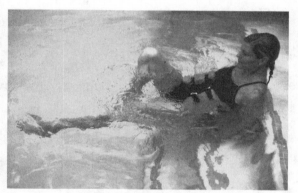

Photo 9-18B. Bicycling on a step.

Power Kicks

Exercises 19 through 21 are especially effective at strengthening your gluteal muscles and other muscles that move the hip. Keep your legs straight the entire time you do them in order to gain the maximum muscular benefit. You will notice that if you engage your core muscles, the exercises are easier to perform, so remind yourself to tighten your abdominals as you begin each one, which will also activate the other core muscles.

No resistance pieces were used on the Speed Kicks because that would have slowed down your ability to focus on speed. Now, as we focus on creating power, you can add resistance pieces when you are ready. How will you know? You will start wishing the exercises were harder so they could be more satisfying. Add Aqualogix Resistance Blades or Hydro-Tone Boots when you get hungry for harder work. (See the appendix at the back of the book.)

Brace yourself at the side of the pool as shown in Photo 9-19A. Lean forward and look down at the water. Let your hips float near the surface of the water, and let your right leg dangle below you as shown. Push your left leg straight back, but not so high as to arch your back. Now switch leg positions and keep reswitching smoothly, taking care to hold your hips steady. Don't let them roll from side to side. Focus on keeping your legs straight and contracting your gluteal muscles to enhance the backward push. Each right-left sequence counts as one repetition. Do twenty reps.

Athletes: Build up quickly to your maximum effort level, and squeeze each side of the buttocks in turn. Squeeze the left buttock when the left leg pushes back and the right buttock when the right leg pushes back. Maintain maximum effort for one minute. Add Aqualogix Resistance Blades or Hydro-Tone Boots when you want to make it harder. (See Photo 9-19B.)

The most common mistake people make on this exercise is to look forward rather than down at the water. That lowers their hips. Keep your hips as high in the water as possible by keeping your eyes focused on the water throughout this exercise.

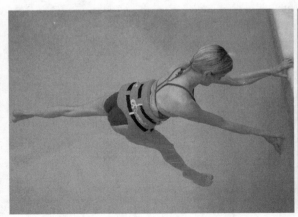

Photo 9-19A. Deep Back Kicks.

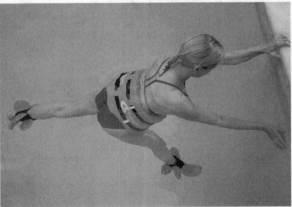

Photo 9-19B. Aqualogix Blades added for resistance.

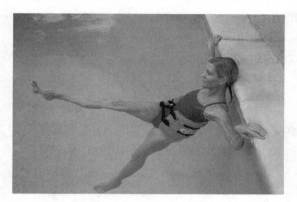

Photo 9-20A. Straight-Leg Deep Kick.

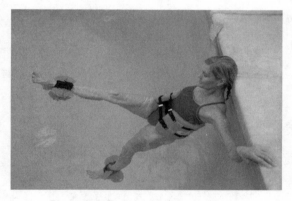

Photo 9-20B. Add Aqualogix Blades
for increased workload.

Brace yourself at the side of the pool as in Photo 9-20A or go to a corner as shown in Photo 9-18A. Your body will float away from the wall if you're wearing a belt, or you might have your back against the wall if you aren't wearing one. Straighten both knees as you lift your right leg to the water's surface, and push your left leg toward the bottom of the pool as shown. Moving with strength, change leg positions so the left leg reaches toward the surface and the right leg sweeps toward the pool bottom. Keep your core muscles engaged throughout the exercise. Do twenty right-left repetitions.

To work your calf muscles at the same time, you can flex the toes up on the foot that lifts and at the same time point the toes down on the foot that drops downward. Say to yourself, "Flex up, point down."

Athletes: Push with maximum effort for one minute. If you don't have a clock to watch, do thirty right-left reps. When you decide you need more resistance, add Aqualogix Resistance Blades or Hydro-Tone Boots.

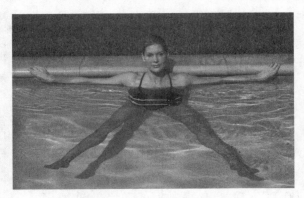

Photo 9-21A. Scissors, Open.

If you're wearing a belt, let your body continue to float slightly away from the pool wall. If you're not wearing a belt, push your lower back against the side of the pool and brace yourself as shown. Open your legs wide as in Photo 9-21A, then touch them together as in Photo 9-21B. Continue opening and closing them, using as much force in opening the legs as you use in closing them. Do twenty reps.

If you're able to cross them, you'll move to the position as in Photo 9-21C. Wait until your hip pain is gone before considering adding resistance pieces as were used in Exercises 19 and 20.

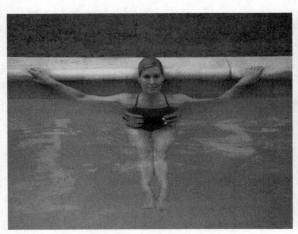

Photo 9-21B. Scissors, Closed.

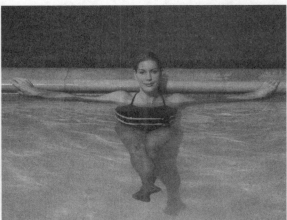

Photo 9-21C. Scissors, Crossed.

Impact Exercises

You can start doing jumping and running exercises in the water long before you can think of doing such movements on land. Usually, jumping up doesn't hurt; it's the landing that causes pain. When you wear a belt, you jump up painlessly; then when you land, the water catches the belt and the belt catches your body, eliminating most of the impact upon landing. Still, we like to start slowly.

Do ten repetitions of the "First Four," Exercises 22 through 25. These are two-legged exercises that give you confidence as you begin adding impact to your program. Don't do more than that the first day. If you don't have pain or discomfort that lasts longer than twenty-four hours, you may perform more impact exercises at your next pool session. If you do have pain that lasts longer than twenty-four hours, you weren't quite ready for these exercises, so you should skip this section and turn to the Lower Body Exercises on page 162. Wait another week or two before trying the First Four again. Aren't you glad you didn't do all thirteen jumping exercises? This is our safety measure. Do *only* the First Four, ten reps. Nothing more.

When you feel good after doing the First Four, you can add a few more impact exercises each time you're in the pool. Do ten reps of each until you're doing ten reps of all the exercises in this section. If one or two exercises cause you pain, skip them, but continue with the rest. Try to add them to your program next week. Over the coming weeks, increase your reps to fifteen for at least two sessions, then increase to twenty reps of all your exercises. Once you've reached twenty reps, start jumping higher to create more workload.

At the same time as you start these jumping exercises, you can begin running as in Exercise 34 on page 160. If running has been a part of your athletic life, you'll find this exhilarating. Perhaps you haven't been able to run for months or even years. But in the water, you can feel the same thrill of pushing hard and getting your heart rate and breathing up to high levels with very little impact on your hip. Follow the suggestions listed or create your own running workout. Increase the running as you increase your reps of the jumps.

The next step is a big one. You've come a long way when you feel confident enough to remove your flotation belt. Start your impact exercises again, this time with only fifteen reps. Skip any exercises that don't feel good to you. You may need to move to slightly deeper water and move a little more slowly in order to feel the same protection you experienced wearing the belt. Trust your own instincts. Put the belt back on if you sense you still need it.

As you gain strength and flexibility in your hip, you might be tempted to return to your normal land activities. Before you do, give your hip and the rest of your body a strong "test drive" in the pool. Find out if your hip is ready for an even greater weight-bearing load on land. Jump high and work hard. Try doing some of the motions of your land activities, such as kicking an imaginary ball against the water's resistance or dancing as you would in a class. If you experience hip pain during or after this test drive, you aren't yet ready to return to land. Continue to prepare your hip for land activities by increasing the number of repetitions you do and by increasing the intensity of your running. You can do thirty reps of each exercise, and you can also add resistance pieces to your power kicks and lower body exercises.

Exercise 22. Lunges

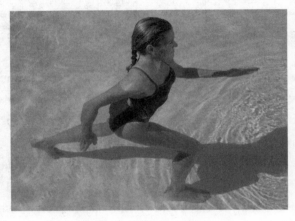

Photo 9-22. Lunges.

Assume the lunge position shown in Photo 9-22 with your right knee forward and bent. Your left leg is straight and to the rear. Your left arm is forward for counterbalance. Jump up and switch arm and leg positions so that the left leg is now forward and the right arm is forward. Make sure your right arm is forward with your left leg and your left arm is forward with your right leg. Each right-left cycle is one repetition.

Exercise 23. Cross Overs or Jacks

Jump to a side-stride position with your legs slightly more than shoulder-width apart, the arms extended out to the sides at water level (Photo 9-23A). Jump again, crossing one arm and leg in front of the other, palms facing in (Photo 9-23B). Return to the starting position, and alternate the arm and leg that cross in front on the cross-over jump. One time your left arm and leg are in front, then on the next rep, your right arm and leg are in front.

If you're uncomfortable or feel hip pain when you cross, you can do the milder version of this exercise called Jacks. In that case, you will begin in the same position as 9-23A, but can simply bring your arms and legs together with your knees bent as in Photo 9-24 A. Use Jacks as a way to begin and then start doing Cross Overs when you can without discomfort. Each open-close or open-cross cycle is one repetition.

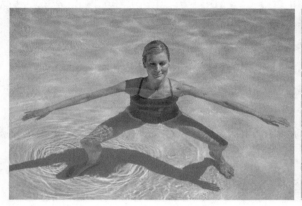

Photo 9-23A. Jacks or Cross Overs.

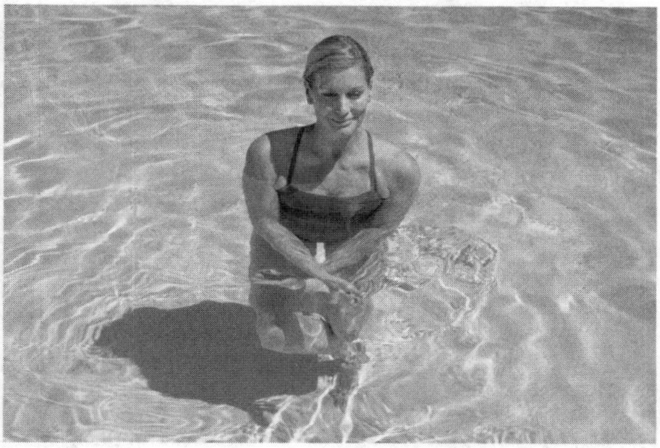

Photo 9-23B. Cross Overs.

Exercise 24. Squat Jumps

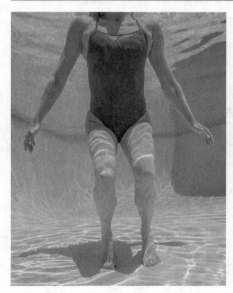

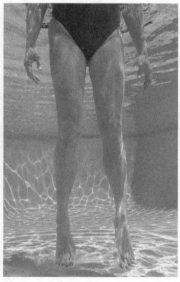

Bend your knees with your feet and knees pointing straight forward as in Photo 9-24A. Jump upward as in Photo 9-24B. As you land, bend your knees to prepare for the next vertical jump. Start with low jumps before trying to jump higher.

Photo 9-24A. Squat Jumps. Also, Jacks.

Photo 9-24B. Squat Jumps.

Exercise 25. Power Frog Jumps

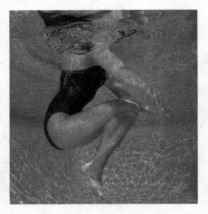

Photo 9-25. Power Frog Jumps.

Bounce gently with your feet together and your arms out to your sides at chest level. Jump off both feet, and lift both knees toward your chest as you sweep both arms forward to meet in front of you as in Photo 9-25. Push the arms back to their starting position as your feet return to the pool bottom. As you begin, you can sit low in the water. As you get stronger, jump higher and pull your hands powerfully to the front.

Exercise 26. Side Straddles

Skip this exercise if you feel pain in your lower back on the first few test jumps.

Begin bouncing with your legs together as in Photo 9-26A. Jump up, open your legs apart (Photo 9-26B), then pull them back together before landing on the pool bottom. Your hands are to your sides for balance. Bend your knees as you land to regain your balance before the next immediate jump. Don't take extra bounces between straddles.

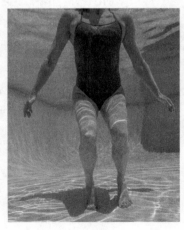

Photo 9-26A. Side Straddles.

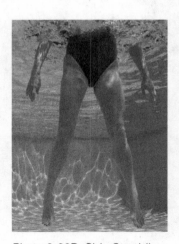

Photo 9-26B. Side Straddles.

HEAL YOUR HIPS

Exercise 27. Front Straddles

Begin bouncing with the legs together as in Photo 9-27A. Jump up and reach the legs into a front split position (Photo 9-27B), and then pull them back together before landing on the pool bottom. Your hands are to your sides for balance. Bend your knees for a soft landing and to allow extra time to regain balance before jumping up with the opposite leg forward in the split position. Each jump equals one repetition.

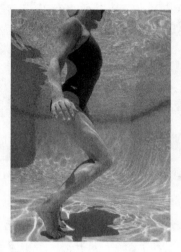

Photo 9-27A. Front Straddles.

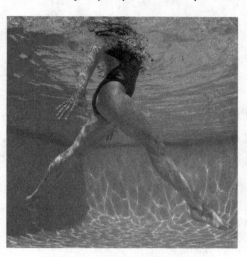

Photo 9-27B. Front Straddles.

Exercise 28. V-Kicks

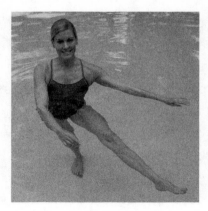

Photo 9-28. V-Kicks.

Stand on your right leg and reach your straight left leg up and out to the side at a 45-degree angle as in Photo 9-28. Now bounce onto your left leg and lift your right leg up to the side, keeping it straight. Sweep both arms toward the leg that lifts. Keep your legs straight throughout this exercise except for the brief moment that the foot touches down and pushes off again. Swinging back and forth is one repetition.

Exercise 29. Double Heel Lifts

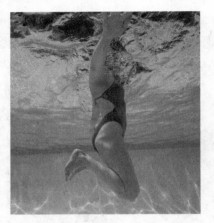

Photo 9-29. Double Heel Lifts.

Bounce with your feet pointing forward, comfortably apart. Use your feet and your toes to push off as you bounce. Now push off and **keep your knees down** while you lift both heels toward your buttocks as in Photo 9-29. Land on both feet and immediately perform the next Double Heel Lift.

Exercise 30. Bouncing Leg Swings

If you feel hip pain as you reach your leg forward, don't lift it so high. If you have hip flexor tendinitis or have been diagnosed with FAI, reach only slightly to the front as per the arrow in Photo 9-30A and emphasize the backward swing. To identify hip flexor tendinitis, press on the front of your thigh at the top where it meets your torso. If you feel a sharp pain, lift your leg gently and see if it increases. Tendinitis is felt primarily when you move. If you have lower back problems, don't swing your leg so far behind you.

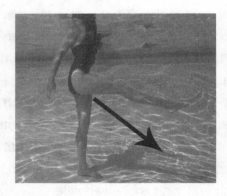

Photo 9-30A. Lift only as high as the arrow if you have FAI or hip flexor tendinitis.

Start bouncing on your stronger leg with your affected leg stretched out in front of you. Hold your opposite arm in front of you to create an opposition position (Photo 9-30B). Bounce only on your strong leg; your affected leg will not touch down. Bounce and swing your affected leg behind you as in Photo 9-30C. Notice that as your leg changes position, the opposite arm accompanies it. Bounce again and swing your leg to the front again, either to the full posistion or the lower posi-tion designated by the arrow. Use this command to help you: "Bounce/forward, Bounce/back, Bounce/forward, Bounce/back." Keep the knee of your swinging leg straight the entire time as it swings forward and back.

After you've performed your repetitions while bouncing on the stronger side, switch to do the same number of reps while bouncing on your affected leg. You may have to move to deeper water or move more slowly in order to do it.

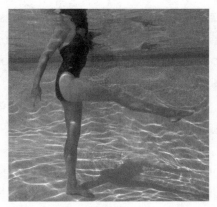

Photo 9-30B. Bouncing Leg Swings.

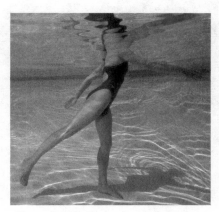

Photo 9-30C. Bouncing Leg Swings.

Exercise 31. Front Kicks

The starting position for this exercise is the same as shown in Photo 9-30A. Lift one leg in front of you with the opposite arm stretched forward for counterbal-ance. Now bounce and switch leg positions so your standing leg is in front and you are now standing on the leg that was in front. Although the legs stay straight as they lift and lower, the knee will bend slightly to allow for the next push-off. Each right-left cycle is one repetition.

Skip this exercise if you feel pain in your lower back on the first few test jumps.

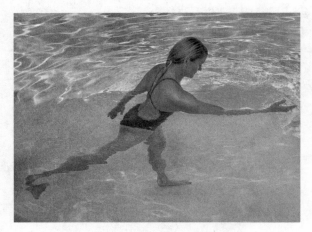

Photo 9-32. Back Kicks.

Assume the position in Photo 9-32. This exercise lets you work the gluteal muscles forcefully while safely strengthening the back muscles. You can place both hands on the side of the pool while you learn this exercise; then move away from the side to use your arms in opposition to your legs as shown.

Stand on your left leg with your right leg straight out behind you. Your right arm is forward and the left is back for counterbalance. Keep your chest forward and your chin down to protect your lower back. Bend your knee, then jump and land on your bent right leg while swinging your straight left leg behind you. Squeeze the gluteal muscles throughout the backward swing. Your left arm is now forward and your right back. Each time you land, bend your knee to lower your chin almost to the water. Keep looking down at the water to maintain the forward position needed to create maximum contraction of the gluteal muscles.

Now jump and land again on your left leg while swinging your straight right leg behind, squeezing the right gluteal. Each right-left cycle is one repetition.

Exercise 33. One-Legged Frog Jumps

Bounce on your stronger leg, and bend the knee of your affected leg in front of you, as in Photo 9-33A. Hold your arms out to your sides for balance. Bounce only on this leg for the first half of the exercise. The other leg won't touch down until you switch sides. Now push off with your weight-bearing leg, and lift that knee up to meet the knee you have been holding in front of you as shown in Photo 9-33B. Then drop your working leg so your foot touches the pool bottom. Immediately bend your knee and prepare for another push-off. Do your repetitions on this leg, then try to duplicate the same pushing and lifting movement with your affected leg. Start by sitting low in the water and barely lifting your knee on the sore side. If your hip feels fine, start pushing off harder and standing taller in the water.

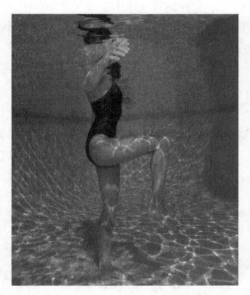

Photo 9-33A. One-Legged Frog Jumps.

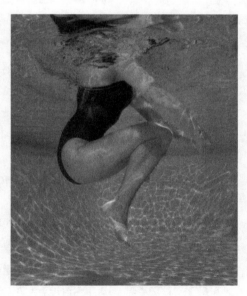

Photo 9-33B. One-Legged Frog Jumps.

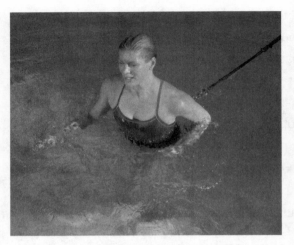

Photo 9-34. Shallow-Water Running with tether.

Begin running in place, simulating good running form on land. (Do not run across the pool because that creates entirely different forces on your body and hip.) The head and chest are erect and the eyes look straight ahead. The shoulders stay down and stable without rocking side to side. As your knees lift, pull your arms directly forward and back without any lateral movement. Make sure you are using opposition: your right arm is forward with your left knee, and your left arm is forward with your right knee.

Once you've established good running form, begin increasing your speed. If your form breaks down, slow down and correct your biomechanics. Then pick up the pace again. When your hip has been pain-free at least two weeks, try these sample intervals. A work period is followed by a slower recovery period, then another work period until you've completed two to five minutes of running. Monitor your heart rate where noted. See the box on page 137 for details on taking your heart rate.

Try the medium-intensity intervals the first session. If they seem too difficult, switch to low intensity right away. If the medium-intensity intervals seem too easy, don't move up to high intensity until the next session. You won't know until later that day or the next day if your muscles or hip are going to be sore or if you will become overly fatigued.

Run in chest-deep water at first, but as you pick up speed, you'll find it easier to run faster in water that is right at the crook of your elbow as seen in Photo 9-34.

Athletes: You don't need a tether to begin. But when you reach top speed, you may find yourself drifting rather than staying in one spot. To be able to apply your full speed to your pool session, tether yourself to a railing, ladder, or other fixture on the side of the pool as in the photo. (See the appendix at the end of the book for more information on the Waterpower Workout Tether.) If you can't find anything to tether to, you can tie a rope to a nearby tree if the pool is outdoors, or ask a training partner to hold the end.

Low-Intensity Program

Run (easy), one to two minutes

Walk across the pool and back

Run (easy), one to two minutes

(Heart-rate check)

Medium-Intensity Program

Run (easy), one minute

Run (medium or fast), thirty seconds

Run (easy), thirty seconds

Run (medium or fast), forty-five seconds

Run (easy), thirty seconds

Run (medium), one minute

(Heart-rate check)

Repeat this sequence if you wish.

High-Intensity Program

Tether yourself to a railing or a ladder on the side of the pool when running at high speeds. This allows you to remain stable and focus on your workload instead of constantly adjusting your position.

Run (easy), thirty seconds

Run (sprint), thirty seconds

(Heart-rate check)

Repeat the above sequence two more times.

Run (easy), thirty seconds

Run (sprint), forty-five seconds

(Heart-rate check)

Repeat this sequence two more times.

Gradually increase the difficulty of your interval session over the next weeks and months. If you are preparing to return to golf, tennis, or other land activities, you can eliminate the deep-water intervals and focus your time and effort on the shallow-water intervals. Use what you've learned about interval training from the examples above to create your own personalized interval session that lasts ten to twenty minutes. Vary it from day to day to avoid losing interest.

Lower Body Exercises

If you feel any pain during these exercises, *slow down or narrow the range of motion.* You'll start your program using only the water's resistance against your legs. As your strength improves, you can add one of the following pieces as your individual needs dictate. Try a Hydro-Fit Buoyancy Cuff if you need buoyancy to increase your hip's range of motion. Start with the mini cuff and progress to the standard cuff over a few weeks. Move slowly as you feel it lift your leg higher than usual. This piece will require more muscular effort as you bring your leg back down to the starting position. After optimal ROM is achieved, transition to the Aqualogix Low-Resistance Blade, then a few weeks later to the High-Resistance Blade. If you still want more workload, use a Hydro-Tone Boot for maximum resistance to increase your strength. (All these pieces are shown in Photo 8-1 on page 116. Details on each are in the appendix.)

Keep in mind that your hip can feel different every day, so you must adjust your workload accordingly. *If your hip is painful, don't use the resistance equipment.* Save the extra resistance for days when your hip and the muscles around it are feeling pain-free and eager for more work.

Notice if your sore hip is weaker than your healthier hip. In that case, you may decide to do more repetitions on the sore side to try to bring it slowly back to equal strength. The easiest way to do more work on one side is to do all your exercises on the sore leg, do a second set on the healthy side, then go back to the sore side for a third set.

Exercise 35. Lateral Leg Raises

Stand with your right hand on the side of the pool facing the end of the pool (Photo 9-35A). Maintain erect posture and lift your left leg directly to the side (Photo 9-35B). Don't lean to the side to be able to lift your leg higher. Keep your feet parallel so that your left knee points forward rather than upward. Pull your left leg back to the starting position. Apply equal force as you lift your leg up and pull it down. Do ten to twenty reps, then turn and repeat with the right leg.

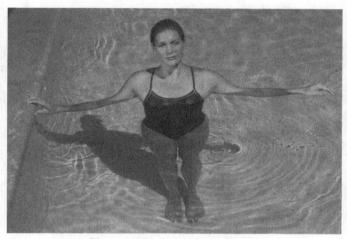

Photo 9-35A. Lateral Leg Raise.

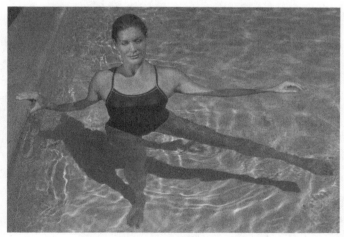

Photo 9-35B. Lateral Leg Raise.

Exercise 36. Leg Swings

To stabilize and protect your lower back, tighten your abdominal and gluteal muscles as you do this exercise.

Continue standing erect with your hand on the side of the pool for stability. Swing your right leg straight forward (Photo 9-36A); then swing it down and to the rear (Photo 9-36B). If a full swing forward hurts your hip, don't reach so far. If a full swing backward hurts your back, don't reach so far. Do ten to twenty reps, then turn and repeat with the right leg.

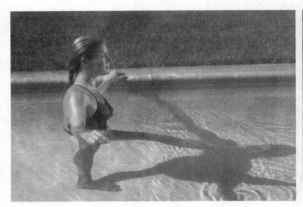

Photo 9-36A. Leg Swings.

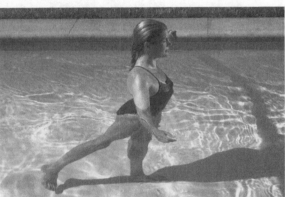

Photo 9-36B. Leg Swings.

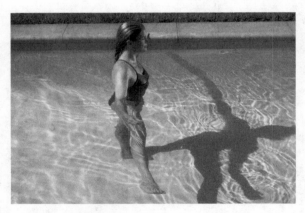

Photo 9-37. Leg Circles. Combine these
three photos as described in Exercise 37.

Exercise 37. Leg Circles

If you have lower back pain, make much smaller circles than shown in the photos mentioned.

Lift your right leg straight forward in front of you just as you began your Leg Swings (Photo 9-36A). This time, however, smoothly sweep your leg in a circular clockwise motion by swinging the leg out to your right side (Photo 9-37), then behind you (Photo 9-36B). Complete the circle by swinging your right leg past your left leg, then beginning the next large circle. Start with five circles in this clockwise direction before doing the same number counter-clockwise. Over the next weeks build up gradually to doing twenty reps in each direction.

Carefully monitor for pain that would tell you either to slow down or make your circles smaller. If you have no such pain, reach as far as you can in each direction. **This is one of your most important exercises in attempting to regain full range of motion of your hip, for only in water can you perform this full circumduction of the hip against a smooth three-dimensional resistance.**

Use these commands: "Front, Side, Back; Front, Side, Back." Do one set of clockwise circles, then a set of counter-clockwise circles. When doing counter-clockwise circles, you'll say the reverse to yourself: "Back, Side, Front, Back, Side, Front." Now turn to do both sets of circles with the other leg.

After you can do smooth, circular motions at an increased range of motion, add an Aqualogix Blade, or a Hydro-Tone Boot to gain maximum strength in this important exercise.

Exercise 38. Knee Swivels

Stand with your right knee bent and your thigh parallel to the surface of the water as in Photo 9-38A. For stability, tighten the muscles of your left leg and buttock. Without moving the rest of your body, swivel your right knee out to the side as in Photo 9-38B. Keep your hips facing forward, and don't use your left leg to rotate your body to the side.

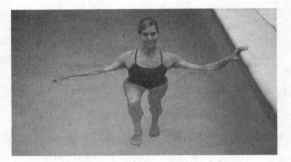

Photo 9-38A. Knee Swivels.

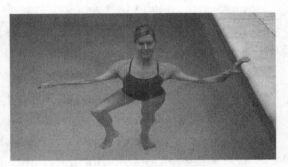

Photo 9-38B. Knee Swivels.

Exercise 39. Four-Way Hip, Three-Way Hip

If you have hip flexor tendinitis or have been diagnosed with FAI, skip this exercise and do only Exercise 40, Two-Way Hip, shown on page 169.

This advanced exercise gives wonderful results for strengthening your core as well as all the muscles surrounding your hip. Learn it by standing on the pool bottom, holding onto the side of the pool. You'll begin without resistance equipment and as you progress, add the Aqualogix Blade shown. As soon as you can, however, you'll want to do it in the freestanding way shown to strengthen your balance and make your hip more stable. Then, if you wish to make it even harder, you can use a step as shown. By standing on a 6-inch or 8-inch step, you lift more of your weight out of the water and therefore have to work harder because you have less support from the water.

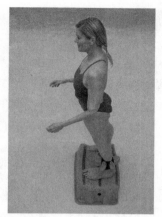

Photo 9-39A. Four-Way Hip. Starting position.

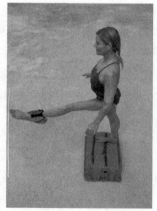

Photo 9-39B. Four-Way Hip, front.

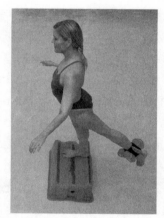

Photo 9-39C. Four-Way Hip, back.

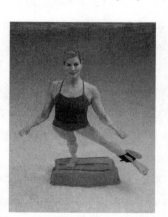

Photo 9-39D. Four-Way Hip, side.

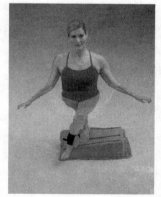

Photo 9-39E. Four-Way Hip, cross.
Eliminate this in 3-Way Hip.

Whether your feet are on the pool bottom or in the middle of a step as shown in Photo 9-39A, find a focal point straight in front of you and keep your eyes focused there. That can make all the difference in maintaining good balance. Engage your core muscles and the muscles in your toes to grasp onto the step or pool bottom. Notice that you will be moving your affected leg in various directions, then returning it to the center position after each movement. That gives you time to regain your balance between each action. Balancing and stabilizing is as important a part of this exercise as is the movement aspect. Start by standing on your stronger leg while you move your affected leg. Then when you switch to stand on your affected leg, try to duplicate the muscular exertion and stability achieved by your stronger leg.

Put all your weight on your unaffected leg and move your affected leg slowly through these motions. First lift your affected leg to the front as high as you can without losing your balance or feeling discomfort. See Photo 9-39B. Bring the leg back to center. Reach the same leg behind you as far as you comfortably can. See Photo 9-39C. Bring the leg back to center. Next lift your affected leg to the side without leaning or letting your hips collapse. See Photo 9-39D. Bring your leg back to center. The final movement is to cross your affected leg in front of your standing leg as in Photo 9-39E. You may decide to eliminate the crossing movement if it causes you pain or discomfort. In that case, you will do a Three-Way Hip exercise rather than Four-Way Hip.

If you do Four-Way Hip, use these commands to remind yourself how to do it: "Front/center, Back/center, Side/center, Cross/center."

For Three-Way Hip, use these commands: "Front/center, Back/center, Side/center."

Now shift all your weight onto your affected leg as you focus your eyes, engage your core muscles, and grasp your toes onto the pool bottom or step. As you move your unaffected leg slowly through these motions, pay great attention to remaining stable on your affected leg.

After a few weeks, when you feel you've mastered this exercise, you can add the minimal resistance Aqualogix Blade. Only when that becomes easy should you consider moving up to the maximum resistance Aqualogix Blade in the photos.

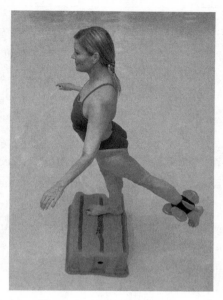

Photo 9-40A. Two-Way Hip.

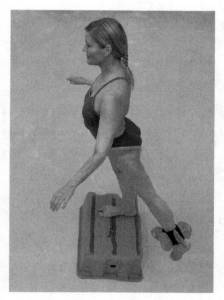

Photo 9-40B. Two-Way Hip.

You can start holding onto the side of the pool for balance, then move away to stand on the pool bottom. When you have mastered the exercise, you can add resistance pieces. When you want to make the exercise harder, use a step as shown.

Keep your eyes on a focal point straight in front of you to help you maintain good balance. Balancing and stabilizing is as important a part of this exercise as is the movement aspect. Engage your core muscles and the muscles in your feet and toes to grasp onto the step or pool bottom. Stand on your stronger leg while you move your affected leg. Then when you switch to stand on your affected leg, try to duplicate the stability exerted by your stronger leg.

Reach your affected leg straight behind you, but only so far as you have pain-free movement. See Photo 9-40A. Keep your attention on squeezing the gluteal muscles to initiate and perform the movement. If you were standing in the center of a clock, you would be reaching your leg back to 6 o'clock. Now, instead of moving your leg to the side, which would be 9 o'clock, you will reach halfway behind the side and the back, between 7 and 8 o'clock as shown in Photo 9-40B.

Now shift all your weight onto your affected leg as you focus your eyes, engage your core muscles, and grasp your toes onto the pool bottom or step. As you move your unaffected leg slowly through these motions pay great attention to remaining stable on your affected leg.

Hip Distraction Technique

This **distraction** technique (pulling in different directions) can be instrumental in reducing or even eliminating your hip pain at the end of the session. Let's say you started the session with moderate, ongoing pain that you feel both day and night. Perhaps during the session you felt a few sharp stabs of pain that subsided as you continued. You worked more slowly with smaller motions when your hip hurt and you pushed against the water's resistance harder when your hip "liked" that particular exercise. That's exactly the way to guide yourself!

The patients in our pool consider this distraction technique their reward for having worked hard during a pool therapy session. They completely relax; some even fall asleep as they suspend motionless in the deep end of the pool with gravity pulling on their ankle weights and their hips. In effect, this is the gentlest traction. It feels good, and you can do it for yourself. Here's how you can enjoy this deeply soothing experience.

What you need:

- The flotation belt you were using earlier in the session.
- An extra belt if you're going to use more than five pounds of weight on each ankle.
- Several pairs of ankle weights to see what feels best—1-lb., 2.5-lb., 5-lb.
- Two Styrofoam noodles.

If you're female, short, and slight, you will probably start with 1-pound or 2.5-pound weights on each ankle. If you're male, tall, and athletic, you should probably start with 5-pound weights on each ankle plus another pair of 2.5-pound weights just above the larger weights on each ankle. Always start light and work your way up. Better that you err on the side of not enough traction and add more next time than create pain from too much weight.

Put on the equipment in this order as you set up for Hip Distraction:

- The belt goes on *first* for safety.
- Use two belts to provide adequate flotation if you're using heavy weights.
- Put on the ankle weights in shallow water, not deep.
- Place the first noodle around your back and under your arms with the loose ends facing forward.

- Put the loose ends of the second noodle under your arms and on top of the first noodle. The middle of the noodle will curve out in front of you.
- If you feel you need more buoyancy because you're using heavy weights, use extra noodles rather than a third belt.
- *Always* remove your ankle weights in the shallow end of the pool before you take off your flotation belt.

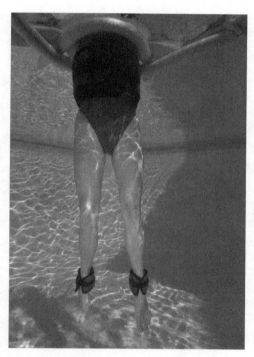

Photo 9-41. Hip Distraction Technique

This comprehensive pool program gives you virtually everything you need for your hip. In the next chapter, you'll learn some variations that are specifically for those who have had either arthroscopic or implant surgery.

10

POSTSURGICAL POOL PROGRAM

If you had hip surgery within the past six months, your pool program will be made from the exercises in this chapter. We will refer back to many of the photos and basic exercises in chapter 9, but this chapter will show you what adjustments need to be made to keep you safe and pain-free as you move through your postsurgical rehabilitation.

KlapperVision: Picture a cook in the kitchen adding a little salt or pepper to taste as he makes spaghetti sauce. Then picture a baker who doesn't veer from the recipe because he doesn't get to taste the cake or modify it during the baking process. Exercising your hip before surgery is a bit like cooking spaghetti sauce—you can try things out and change what you're doing based on what you feel. But exercising your hip after surgery is more like baking a cake—you need to know what ingredients should be part of your exercise regimen and what shouldn't.

After surgery, the wound is healing, as are the internal repairs that your surgeon made. You need someone to guide you who has gone before you and created a plan for recovery. With correct guidance, you'll feel safe making appropriate movements and you won't do inappropriate motions that could damage your healing hip. While our protocol for implant surgery has proven successful over many decades, the protocols for the new FAI and labral repair surgeries continue to change, as does the rehabilitation process. This is why **we recommend that your arthroscopic hip surgeon be a partner in planning your postoperative recovery**. Writing a prescription for physical therapy isn't enough. The repairs inside your hip are biologic, meaning your own tissue is being repaired, not replaced by metal. This presents many variables, so a conversation between your therapist and surgeon is in order. Your therapist will want to know what the doctor found in surgery and if there is anything for which you might be at risk. Most relevant, the therapist needs to know if he can be aggressive or not. Each program must be individualized. Only the surgeon knows exactly what happened inside your hip joint, and he knows if there's any reason to be cautious. For instance, the therapist would be asked not to be aggressive if the labral repair was tenuous, meaning it wasn't very sturdy. But if the labrum was completely repaired in its full consistency, your therapist might be told when he could start being more aggressive.

Those of you who learned this program prior to surgery will smile at the thought of resuming your pool program. You already know how to balance in the deep-water intervals, and you've learned good form on all the other exercises. They have become second nature to your body. Now you can apply the skill you acquired and not be nervous about getting into the pool. If you're finding this book only after surgery, don't worry. We'll guide you through all the exercises with expert care.

Your surgeon will tell you when you are allowed to enter the water. We allow our arthroscopy patients to get in the pool after two weeks and the implant patients after four weeks. Arthroscopy patients should follow this guideline: from two weeks to six weeks, focus on using the buoyancy of the water to gain range of motion, then start building strength after the six-week mark.

Hip Implant Patients

Get your surgeon's approval before beginning any new exercise program. Check with your physical therapist if you have concerns or questions about specific exercises.

Call me old-fashioned—I still ask my patients to follow the precautions below. Even if your doctor says you have no movement precautions after your surgery, you can be more comfortable and not disrupt the systematic formation of good scar tissue by following these precautions *whether you were told you need them or not.* You don't have to reach for full motion right away just because you were told you could.

Hip Precautions

- Do not let your knee or ankle cross the midline of your body.
- Avoid hip flexion of more than 90 degrees.
- Don't combine hip flexion with internal rotation (see Photo 15-1, page 285).
- When you reach the side of the pool after walking across it, always turn away from your postsurgical side to keep from forcing that hip into internal rotation (see Photo 15-2, page 285).
- If you drop your soap in the shower after your therapy session, do not bend to pick it up.

—Robert Klapper, MD

Gait Training

Read the introductory material on page 128 about the purpose of gait training, which is to regain a strong, normalized walking pattern. Read the helpful hints and learn how to do the techniques that start on page 129. Your normal walking pattern will have to be rebuilt with the following exercises. Spend extra time on gait training until an observer—a training partner, coach, or aquatic therapist—says you are walking normally again.

A Helpful Visualization

Some patients have had bad gait patterns for so many years that they feel quite normal lurching from side to side as they walk. Even in chest-deep water they limp badly and can't quite conceptualize what a normal gait would be. Try this visualization: Pretend that the sides of your body are made of steel and that a bell hangs straight down the center of your body from a string attached to your head. If you lean to the right, the bell will clang noisily against the right steel wall, and if you lean to the left, it will clang against the left steel wall. Do everything in your power to keep that imaginary bell hanging straight down from your head, not swinging from side to side.

Here's a chance to start using your mental power to enhance your movements. It all starts in the mind.

Exercise 1. Shallow-Water Walking—Backward, Forward, Sideways

(See page 129.)

Recovering from hip arthroscopy: Hip pain may have altered your normal walking pattern prior to surgery. Although the presurgical pain may have been eliminated, you could be surprised to find that you are still limping. If this is the case, your limp is just a bad habit, and it's time to break it.

Recovering from hip implant surgery: Use a pool with a relatively unslanted bottom. If the pool is steeply slanted, you'll find yourself walking with one leg functionally longer than the other. You don't want that, so drive the extra few miles to a pool that will provide you with a level pool bottom.

When walking across the pool, turn away from your postsurgical leg. That way you won't inadvertently turn your leg into internal rotation. (See Photo 15-2, page 285.) For example, if you had surgery on your right hip, always turn to your left when you reach the side of the pool.

Exercise 2. Marching

(See page 130.)

Recovering from hip arthroscopy: Lift your knee to only 45 degrees—half as high as the 90 degrees shown in Photo 9-2 on page 130. Maintain this low knee lift for the first six weeks after surgery.

Recovering from hip implant surgery: Lift your knee to only 45 degrees—half as high as the 90 degrees shown in Photo 9-2 on page 130. Over the weeks and months your knee will begin to rise up toward 90 degrees by itself. Don't force it. Do not let your knee cross the midline of the body.

Exercise 3. Long-Leg Walk

(See page 131.)

Recovering from hip arthroscopy: Skip this exercise until three months after FAI surgery. Get your surgeon's approval before you start it. When you do, lift your leg very gently to the front, starting with only 45 degrees. If you are pain-free, you can gradually lift it higher over the next months. If you have hip flexor tendinitis, avoid this exercise. To identify hip flexor tendinitis, press on the front of your thigh at the top where it meets your torso. If you feel a sharp pain, lift your leg gently and see if it increases. Tendinitis is felt primarily when you move.

Recovering from hip implant surgery: Skip this exercise until all the other Gait Training Exercises have become easy and you are walking without a limp. When you add it, move slowly and lift each leg only as high as you comfortably can. Over time the leg will start lifting higher without your having to force it.

Deep-Water Intervals

If you already learned to do the techniques that make up Deep-Water Intervals, you'll start this section with inner confidence. If this is new to you, or if you feel tentative about doing these deep-water techniques, you can start your warm-up holding on to the pool for stability as show in Photo 10-4. You can do your entire series of low-level intervals in this same position. Once you've gained enough confidence to move away from the side of the pool, you'll benefit from increased core and upper body strength as you add arm movements in coordination with the leg movements.

Hip arthroscopy and implant patients can do Exercises 4 through 6 as soon as they are cleared to enter the pool after surgery. If this is a new program for you, be prepared for a thrill as you can run and walk without any weight on your hip at all!

Exercise 4. Deep-Water Running

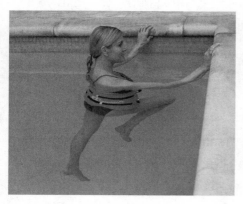

Photo 10-4.
Deep-Water Running in corner.

(See page 132.)

Don't lift your knees as high as the 90 degrees shown in Photo 10-4. Start gradually, barely lifting one knee and then the other, stopping at the level at which you feel comfortable. Keep your knees pointing straight forward. Don't let your knees turn in, crossing the midline of the body.

Exercise 5. Deep-Water Walking—Basic Walk and Power Walk

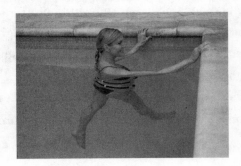

Photo 10-5.
Deep-Water Walking in corner.

(See page 134.)

Stick with the basic walking maneuver for the first two to three weeks. Very gradually introduce Power Walk into your program, but if you feel undue strain in the hip flexors, quads, or hamstrings, return to the Basic Walk and try again next week.

In performing any of the walking motions, put your attention on your gluteal muscles. Try to initiate each backward pull with a gluteal muscle contraction. If you take your mind off this, you won't get as much gluteal strengthening from the movement.

Exercise 6. Flies

(See pages 134–135.)

Recovering from hip arthroscopy: Start by gently doing the original version shown in Photos 9-6A and 9-6B on pages 134–135. Once you can balance and stay in one place as you do it, try the variation that follows. **You want to emphasize the internal rotation as you touch your big toes together as in Photo 10-6.1B. You have the first six weeks after surgery to regain your internal rotation, so take this exercise seriously.**

Recovering from hip implant surgery: Some orthopedic surgeons allow their patients to perform abduction and adduction (opening and closing) of the hips within two weeks of surgery. Different surgical techniques and implants require different postsurgical practices, so ask your doctor when you can begin this exercise.

Exercise 6.1. Flies Variation, External Rotation and Internal Rotation

If you had implant surgery, get your doctor's permission before doing this exercise.

Continue doing Flies. As you reach your arms and legs out to the sides, externally rotate your hips, which means that your feet and your toes point outward as in Photo 10-6.1A. As you return your arms and legs to center, internally rotate your hips and touch your big toes together as in Photo 10-6.1B. Use these commands to coach yourself through it: "Toes out on the way out; toes in on the way in."

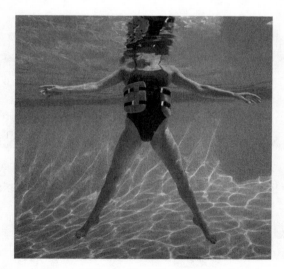

Photo 10-6.1A. Flies, External Rotation.

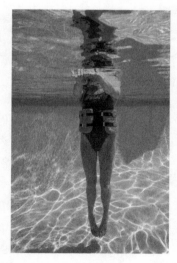

Photo 10-6.1B. Flies, Internal Rotation.

Exercise 7. Speed Walk

(See page 136.)

Recovering from hip arthroscopy: Wait until three months after surgery to do this exercise. Get your surgeon's approval before trying it. It's a lot harder than it looks. You need to be well coordinated and strong enough to move quickly to perform it correctly. If the quick movements cause you deep hip pain, slow down. Over the next weeks and months you can gradually increase your speed and effort level.

Recovering from hip implant surgery: Wait until six weeks after surgery to try this exercise. You'll want to work on developing good core, hip flexor, and gluteal muscle strength before you start this fast-action exercise that uses all of those muscles in rapid succession. If the quick movements cause you deep hip pain, slow down. Over the next weeks and months you can increase your effort level and speed.

Exercise 8. Deep-Water Intervals (DWIs)

(See page 136.)

Recovering from hip arthroscopy: Do the low-intensity program the first four weeks after surgery, then progress to the medium-intensity program. If you feel undue pain in your hip from increasing the speed of movement, return to the low-intensity program for another two weeks before trying to progress again. Use that same rule of thumb in another month if you wish to progress to the high-intensity program.

Recovering from hip implant surgery: Do the low-intensity program for the first six weeks after surgery. When this program starts to feel too easy, try the medium-intensity program. If you feel undue pain in your hip from increasing the speed of movement, return to the low-intensity program for another two weeks before trying to progress again. Use that same rule of thumb in another few months if you wish to progress to the high-intensity program.

Stretching

Read the introduction to stretching on page 139.

If you had arthroscopic hip surgery, you can begin all the stretches at the two-week mark or when your surgeon allows you to enter the water. If you had implant surgery, your doctor may have you wait four weeks or more to make sure your incision is super sealed.

Start each stretch very gently. Back away from any pain you may feel by releasing the stretch to a comfortable position.

Exercise 9. Hamstring Stretch

(See page 140.)

Lift your leg to only 45 degrees (lower on the wall than in Photo 9-9 on page 140), and bend your knee slightly if you must. Do not lean your head or chest forward. Maintain a focal point straight in front of you so that your head and chest will be upright. You can gradually move your foot higher as the weeks pass.

Exercise 10. Body Swing

(See page 141.)

Start swinging gently from side to side in a controlled fashion. Don't try to push deeply into this stretch until after the six-week mark.

Exercise 11. Lateral Split

(See page 141.)

Recovering from hip implant surgery: Some surgeons ask you not to do hip abduction (opening of the legs) during the first weeks after surgery. Other surgeons want you to do hip abduction right away to start strengthening those muscles, which are the hip stabilizers. Ask your surgeon when you can begin doing this exercise. When you add it, place your feet lower on the wall than the position shown in Photo 9-11 on page 141. Very gently open your legs comfortably apart. Do not force this stretch, and do not lean forward for at least six weeks.

Exercise 12. Quad Stretch

(See page 142.)

Recovering from hip implant surgery: You may not be able to assume the position in Photo 9-12 for several months after surgery. In that case, you can put a strap around your foot and pull the strap over your shoulder in order to do a quad stretch. If you have an aquatic therapist, he can lift your foot until you can hold it with your hand. We want you to be able to do this stretch, because it's a setup for the next exercise, Hip Flexor Stretch, which is crucial to regaining normal range of motion in your hip.

Exercise 13. Hip Flexor Stretch

(See page 142.)

Recovering from hip arthroscopy: Try this stretch gently at first. If you have undue pain, wait two weeks before trying again.

Recovering from hip implant surgery: Once you can reach the position in Photo 9-12, hold it right there. Don't let your knee drift backward toward the position shown in Photo 9-13 until you get your therapist's or surgeon's permission. When you do, move slowly and carefully and release the position immediately if you feel any undue pain or discomfort.

Deep-Water Exercises

Exercises 14 through 16 are primarily used in non-surgical hips in an attempt to regain full range of motion and avoid or postpone surgery. You can skip this section entirely, or if you wish to try these exercises, wait until six weeks after surgery. Before adding each of these exercises, get permission from your doctor or therapist. You may feel a pinching sensation as you cross your knee or leg in front of your body as in Exercises 14 and 15. If so, wait a few more weeks.

Exercise 14. Bent-Knee Twists

(See page 143.)

Wait at least six weeks before gently trying this exercise.

Exercise 15. Straight-Leg Twists

(See page 144.)

Recovering from hip arthroscopy: Wait until three months after surgery to try this exercise, and if you do, move through a narrow range of motion. Skip this completely if you have hip flexor tendinitis. If the pain resolves and you wish to try this exercise, start slowly, lifting each leg gently against the water's resistance. Focus on pushing the opposite leg down to enhance the gluteal muscle contraction.

Exercise 16. V-Kicks

(See page 144.)

Recovering from hip arthroscopy: Wait until three months after surgery before trying this exercise, and then don't lift your leg as high as seen in Photo 9-16. Skip this completely if you have hip flexor tendinitis. If the pain resolves and you wish to try this exercise, start slowly, lifting each leg gently against the water's resistance. Focus on pushing the opposite leg down to enhance the gluteal muscle contraction.

Kicking Series

As you start the kicking series, move slowly with control. Forget about the Speed Kicks and Power Kicks discussed on page 145 to 147. Treat all the kicks the same, as a wonderful way to strengthen your buttocks, thighs, core muscles, and lower back. They can be a lot of fun at a time when you might be wishing for more fun in your life. If you did the Kicking Series prior to surgery, you may have built up to a high intensity. It's time to start over. Start slowly and each week add a little more force and speed. Don't hurt your hip trying to do too much too soon just for the exhilaration. That can wait as you regain balanced strength between your gluteal muscles and hip flexor muscles.

About a month into your pool rehab, read the section on pages 145 to 147 about Speed Kicks and Power Kicks and implement this into your program. Start increasing the speed of Exercises 17 and 18, and add resistance pieces to Exercises 19 through 21. If you do this too soon, your hip will tell you, so always try anything new with great care the first day. You can always pick up the speed or add more resistance tomorrow.

Exercise 17. Back Flutter Kicks

(See page 146.)

Recovering from hip arthroscopy: Wait six weeks before doing any flutter kicking, either as shown at the side of the pool or in swimming. When you start this exercise, keep your feet below the surface for the first week or two. Focus on using your gluteal muscles on each downstroke.

Recovering from hip implant surgery: As you begin, don't force your feet to break the surface of the water. Your legs will probably feel more comfortable working below the water.

Exercise 18. Bicycling

(See page 147.)

Recovering from hip arthroscopy: You can begin this exercise as soon as your surgeon allows you to go into the pool. Start slowly, and when you feel like increasing your speed, do so gradually.

Recovering from hip implant surgery: As you begin, don't lift your knees above 90 degrees. In fact, your knees may not even break the surface of the water. Over the months, your knee lift will naturally increase. Don't force it.

Exercise 19. Deep Back Kicks

(See page 148 and Photo 9-19A.)

Put your mental power to work by thinking about squeezing the gluteal muscles as each leg pushes backward. Squeeze the left buttock as the left leg reaches back, and squeeze the right buttock as the right leg reaches back. Pay attention to any difference you feel between the two buttocks and work toward building equal strength in each. Use these commands to coach yourself: "Squeeze left, squeeze right, squeeze left, squeeze right."

Recovering from hip arthroscopy: You can do the basic exercise shown in Photo 9-19A as soon as you can enter the pool. Wait until the six-week mark after surgery to consider adding the resistance pieces shown in Photo 9-19B.

Recovering from hip implant surgery: Start with a narrow range of motion at first by minimizing the backward push. Even though you may not have any postsurgical precautions, you will be most comfortable and will help the tissues to heal without disruption if you avoid extremes of flexion (forward bending) and extension (backward reaching) for the first six weeks.

About a month into your pool rehab program, you can consider adding the resistance pieces around your ankles as shown in Photo 9-19B.

Exercise 20. Straight-Leg Deep Kicks

(See page 149.)

Recovering from hip arthroscopy: You can do the basic exercise shown in Photo 9-20A as soon as you can enter the pool. Get your therapist's or surgeon's approval before adding the resistance pieces as shown in Photo 9-20B. They may have you wait as long as three months. *If you have hip flexor tendinitis, do not add resistance.*

Recovering from hip implant surgery: Start with a narrow range of motion at first. Don't reach as far as shown in Photo 9-20A. About a month into your pool rehab program, you can consider adding the resistance pieces around your ankles as shown in Photo 9-20B.

Exercise 21. Scissors, Crossing or No Crossing

(See page 150.)

Recovering from hip arthroscopy: During the first two weeks you're in the pool, perform this exercise slowly. Ask your doctor or therapist if you can cross your legs or not as in Photo 9-21C on page 150. During weeks three and four, gradually apply more force as you push against the water. If you have no undue pain, you can gradually increase the speed and power of the exercise. *Six weeks after your surgery, you can consider adding the resistance pieces shown in Photo 10-21, but not before.*

Recovering from hip implant surgery: Ask your doctor or therapist when you can begin this exercise. Over the weeks you will find your legs naturally floating to a wider and wider position, so don't feel you have to force them. Your range of motion will automatically increase as you continue your pool program and your hip heals from the surgery.

You may have precautions not to cross your surgical leg past the midline of your body, or you might simply find it more comfortable not to cross your legs. In that case, don't cross your legs as you begin this exercise. You can bring your ankles and knees together so they are touching and return to the open position. But we don't want you to become bored, so we've added these two variations.

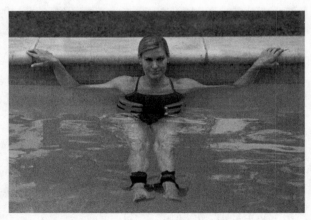

Photo 10-21. Scissors with Aqualogix Blades.

Exercise 21.1. Scissors, No Crossing Variation—Flex Out, Point In

Continue to brace yourself on the side of the pool. As you open your legs, lift up your toes, flexing your feet as in Photo 10-21.1A. As you bring your legs together again, point your toes as in Photo 10-21.1B. By adding this variation, you strengthen your calf muscles, an important muscle group in walking. Use these commands to coach yourself through this exercise: "Flex out, point in, flex out, point in."

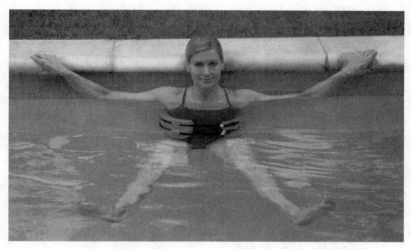

Photo 10-21.1A. Scissors, Feet Flexed.

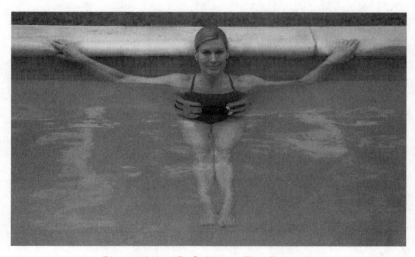

Photo 10-21.1B. Scissors, Feet Pointed.

Recovering from hip arthroscopy: Here's another opportunity to focus on regaining your internal rotation. Do this exercise diligently every time you're in the pool, starting the first day you're in the water.

Recovering from hip implant surgery: Skip this variation for at least six weeks. You don't need to stress all the tissues from the joint capsule up to the skin that are healing.

This time as you open your legs, rotate your hips outward so that your toes point toward the ends of the pool as in Photo 10-21.2A. As you pull your legs together, rotate your hips inward so that your big toes touch as in Photo 10-21.2B.

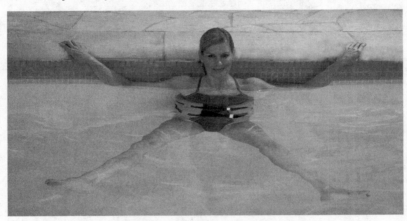

Photo 10-21.2A. Scissors, External Rotation.

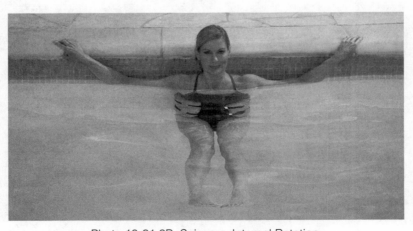

Photo 10-21.2B. Scissors, Internal Rotation.

Impact Exercises

Read the material carefully from page 151 to 152 that explains how to start doing the Impact Exercises safely. You'll see we have a detailed system that allows you to take small steps forward for a safe progression. You'll start doing these exercises in chest-deep water *wearing a flotation belt.* Even if you have to wait a few weeks to find or buy the belt, *don't begin them without it. Your belt is your safety cushion.* You'll start by gently bouncing up and down, learning the rhythm of each exercise. As you master them and gain confidence in your resilience against this gentle impact, you'll start jumping higher. Don't rush this process. Be careful and don't force yourself to do anything that makes you too nervous.

You can move to deeper water if you want less impact, or you can move to shallower water for more stability. Each session you can move to slightly deeper or shallower water to find the right amount of impact that feels good to you but also offers enough stability.

As you do each exercise, put your attention on using your gluteal muscles upon landing. For example, let's look at Exercise 22 on page 152, Lunges. Every time you land, you're stabilizing your pelvis, which is exactly how the gluteal muscles work—you are training your gluteal muscles in their primary function: stabilization. Keep focusing on your gluteal muscles as you do all the Impact Exercises. Research shows that adding your mental power to your muscle power offers greater physical results.

Follow the plan on page 151 in which you will do only ten repetitions of the First Four, Exercises 22 through 25. You can lightly push off, and as you gently land, the water catches your belt and the belt catches most of your weight. You will find yourself smiling. These exercises are *fun*! But don't get carried away. You need to follow the plan of restraint that is offered in chapter 9 to safely get all the exercises into your rehab program. If they cause you any discomfort as you first try them or later that evening, wait a week and try the First Four again.

After you're doing twenty reps of all the exercises, you can remove your flotation belt and congratulate yourself. You've regained important movement skills and capability. The first day you do the Impact Exercises without your float belt, do the right thing—cut back to fifteen reps of each the first day. If you don't have any pain or discomfort, you can go back to twenty reps the next week.

Recovering from hip arthroscopy: *Wait until you are six weeks past surgery before attempting to add these exercises to your program.* Focus on using your gluteal muscles to stabilize your pelvis with each landing.

Recovering from hip implant surgery: Don't begin the Impact Exercises until you've mastered everything else in the program without increasing your hip pain. These are jumping and running exercises and should be introduced after the midpoint in your rehab program.

Exercise 22. Lunges

(See page 152.)

Exercise 23. Cross Overs or Jacks

(See pages 152-153.)

Start by doing Jacks when you first enter the pool after surgery. This means you'll jump to a wide position as in jumping jacks, and jump your feet back together and bend your knees. Your arms will open and close with your legs. You don't need to challenge your hip by crossing your legs right away. Get used to the pool and the exercises, then you can switch from doing Jacks to Cross Overs when you're looking for more of a challenge. Both variations are shown on page 153.

Exercise 24. Squat Jumps

(See page 153.)

Exercise 25. Power Frog Jumps

(See page 154.)

Don't lift your knees as high as shown in Photo 9-25 on page 154. Lift them only as high as you feel you can with confidence and comfort. Over time your knees will naturally start lifting higher as your hip heals.

Exercise 26. Side Straddles

(See page 154.)

If you have an unstable sacroiliac joint, skip this exercise for a few weeks. When you do try it, open your legs only half as wide as you see in Photo 9-26B on page 154. If you don't experience increased pain, you can keep this exercise in your program.

Exercise 27. Front Straddles

(See page 155.)

Recovering from hip implant surgery: Depending on your doctor's surgical approach, you may or may not have extremely tight hip flexor muscles. If you do, you'll find this exercise difficult to do at first. Don't try to reach as far back as shown in Photo 9-27B on page 155 or you're likely to bend your knee significantly. Instead, try to keep your legs straight, even if you open your stride by only six inches. By focusing on straight legs, you'll gain hip extension—the ability to reach your surgical leg behind you.

Exercise 28. V-Kicks

(See page 155.)

Exercise 29. Double Heel Lifts

(See page 156.)

Exercise 30. Bouncing Leg Swings

(See page 156.)

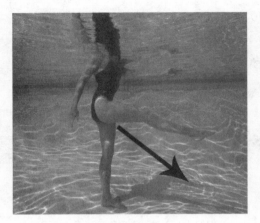

Photo 10-30.
Bouncing Leg Swings, modified.

Recovering from hip arthroscopy: Bounce on your non-surgical leg. Don't reach your surgical leg to the full position shown in Photo 9-30A. Rather, lift your leg only to the height of the arrow in Photo 10-30. Focus on the backswing half of this exercise while you maintain this reduced front swing. Once you've learned the rhythm of the exercise, try it bouncing on your surgical leg. Say to yourself, "Bounce, front. Bounce, back."

Recovering from hip implant surgery: Start by bouncing on your non-surgical leg as you keep your surgical leg straight and swing it comfortably forward and backward with each bounce. You don't have to try to reach the full position forward and backward right away. You will naturally start reaching higher in both directions as your hip heals and you get stronger.

Exercise 31. Front Kicks

(See page 157.)

Exercise 32. Back Kicks

(See page 158.)

This is a great exercise for gluteal strengthening, so be sure to keep this one in your program. If you can't quite figure it out from the still photos, you can see it in action on *Lynda Huey's Waterpower Workout* video. See the appendix on page 323.

HEAL YOUR HIPS

Exercise 33. One-Legged Frog Jumps

(See page 159.)

Exercise 34. Shallow-Water Running

(See page 160.)

Once you begin, do the low-intensity intervals for the first two weeks. When this program starts to feel too easy for both you and your hip, try the medium-intensity intervals. If you feel undue pain in your hip from increasing the speed of movement, return to low intensity for another two weeks before trying to progress again. Use that same rule of thumb in another month or two if you wish to progress to the high-intensity intervals.

Recovering from hip arthroscopy: Don't add Shallow-Water Running to your program until six weeks after surgery. Get your surgeon's or therapist's approval.

Recovering from hip implant surgery: Running in chest-deep water can be added near the middle of your rehab program.

Lower Body Exercises

Read the introductory information about lower body exercises on page 162. You won't use equipment as you start, just the buoyancy and resistance of the water against your legs as you move them. Many people who have had hip surgery will need to use the buoyancy cuffs to regain their normal range of motion (ROM). See Photos 10-35A and 10-35B on page 195. There is a mini and a standard buoyancy cuff. Larger men usually start with the standard, but most others start with the mini and after a few weeks transition to the standard cuff, which has about three times more buoyancy. Work slowly as you get used to the cuffs—although they help you lift your leg, they make it harder for you to pull your leg toward the pool bottom.

After you've regained your normal ROM, you can switch to a resistance blade around your ankle. If your ROM is normal, you'll skip using the buoyancy cuffs and add the resistance pieces to build strength. These pieces are found in the appendix on page 323. Start with the minimal resistance blades, then transition to the maximal resistance blades. That may be the correct amount of resistance for you from now on. If you're feeling strong or wanting a challenge, you can try the Hydro-Tone Boot as shown in Photos 10-36A and 10-36B.

Recovering from hip arthroscopy: You will probably be allowed in the water around two weeks after surgery. You can start all of these easy range-of-motion exercises as soon as you're in the water. Focus on improving your ROM for the first six weeks by using the buoyancy of the water. After six weeks, get your doctor's approval to start using buoyancy cuffs to regain ROM and resistance to create strength gains.

Recovering from hip implant surgery: Use the buoyancy of the water to improve your range of motion. Assuming your non-surgical hip has normal ROM, you'll want to match that with your surgical hip. Once that has happened, you can switch to resistance pieces to work on strength.

Exercise 35. Lateral Leg Raises

(See page 163.)

When you add the buoyancy cuff shown, here's a tip: Initiate the movement by contracting your gluteal muscles. When your leg reaches its maximum height, pause for a moment. Let the buoyancy cuff do its job of lifting just a little more. Then focus on your adductor (inner thigh) muscles, which will have to work harder than before because they are pulling a buoyant cuff toward the bottom of the pool.

Recovering from hip arthroscopy: Get your doctor's or therapist's approval to do this exercise. Also ask when you can begin using the buoyancy cuffs.

Recovering from hip implant surgery: Ask your doctor or therapist when you can begin this exercise. When you first begin it, don't lift your leg very high to the side, and don't use any equipment. A few pool sessions later, you can add the mini buoyancy cuff. If that seems too easy, wait one more session to add the standard buoyancy cuff. Over the next weeks and months you'll find your leg naturally lifting higher and higher almost by itself.

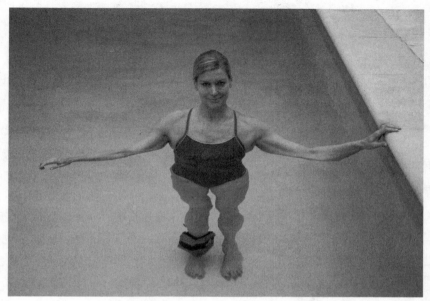

Photo 10-35A. Lateral Leg Raises.

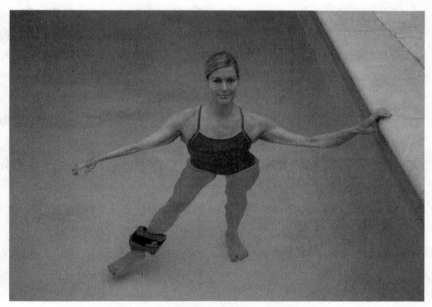

Photo 10-35B. Lateral Leg Raises.

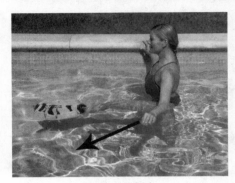

Photo 10-36A.
Leg Swing Forward with
Hydro-Tone Boot.

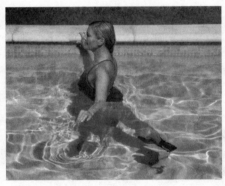

Photo 10-36B.
Leg Swing to Big Toe Touch at
rear with Hydro-Tone Boot.

(See page 164.)

If you have back pain, limit your swing backward by touching your big toe to the floor and no further. See Photo 10-36B.

Start with no equipment. The Hydro-Tone Boot shown in the photos is the final stage in your recovery. Start by using only the buoyancy of the water as you work to regain your range of motion (ROM). Then you'll progress to buoyancy pieces shown in Photos 10-35A and 10-35B. Once you have reestablished your normal ROM, switch to using resistance equipment to gain strength. Start with the Aqualogix Minimum Resistance Blade, then a few weeks later move to the Maximum Resistance Blade. That may feel like the right amount of resistance to you. If you're strong and need more of a challenge, use the Hydro-Tone Boot shown in Photos 10-36A and 10-36B.

Recovering from hip arthroscopy: Use the buoyancy of the water to work on gentle range of motion. Lift your postsurgical leg only as high as the arrow in Photo 10-36A. Emphasize the backswing to increase gluteal strength. When the pain has been gone a few weeks, ask your surgeon or therapist if you can add a buoyancy cuff to gain range of motion. When you have good range, add the resistance pieces next to gain strength.

Recovering from hip implant surgery: As you begin, lift your postsurgical leg only as high as the arrow shown in Photo 10-36A. Limit your backswing as well, as shown in Photo 10-36B. Over the next weeks and months your leg will naturally start lifting higher by itself. Don't force it. Eventually you'll find yourself using your full range of motion.

Exercise 37. Leg Circles

(See pages 164-165.)

Keep your leg low as you start Leg Circles. You can draw your circles with your foot on the pool bottom to get started, then over the next weeks gradually lift your leg toward 45 degrees.

Recovering from hip arthroscopy: Move slowly and gently through a comfortable range of motion. Be sure to do circles in both a clockwise and counter-clockwise direction. Use the waters buoyancy to increase your ROM. After six weeks ask your doctor or therapist if you can add resistance to this motion, and if so, how high you should ideally lift your leg.

Recovering from hip implant surgery: For the first few weeks your hip could be sore. In that case, limit the range of motion. Never force it; let the water float your leg higher and higher naturally over the next weeks and months. When the pain has been gone a few weeks, try adding a buoyancy cuff to gain range of motion. When you have full range, add the resistance pieces next to gain strength.

Exercise 38. Knee Swivels

(See page 166.)

If you find it uncomfortable to do this exercise, drop your knee three to six inches from what is shown in Photo 9-38 and try again.

Recovering from hip arthroscopy: You can start this around the two-week mark when you enter the pool. Smoothly move your hip through a range of motion that feels easy. Don't push it yet. Your doctor will tell you if he wants you to start being more aggressive.

Recovering from hip implant surgery: You may not have great range of motion as you start this exercise, but expect improvements as you continue.

Exercise 39. Four-Way Hip, Three-Way Hip

(See pages 166 to 168.)

Start this exercise holding on to the side of the pool for balance. You will begin to build great stability in your standing leg. When you gain confidence, step away from the side of the pool to do your repetitions. When that gets easy, implant patients can add buoyancy to get full ROM, then add resistance to regain strength. To make it more challenging, stand on a step as in Photos 9-39A to 9-39E.

Recovering from hip arthroscopy: Skip this exercise and do Two-Way Hip instead. See Exercise 40.

Recovering from hip implant surgery: Do Three-Way Hip as you begin, which eliminates the crossing motion that could be uncomfortable for you. If you wish to progress to doing Four-Way Hip, get your therapist's or surgeon's permission first.

If you're having trouble regaining your normal ROM, you can add a buoyancy cuff as you do the exercise. It will lift your leg higher than your normal ROM, at which point you should pause for a second or two. Let the cuff lift your leg and stretch the hip joint. Then return to the starting position.

Exercise 40. Two-Way Hip

(See pages 169-170.)

Start this exercise holding on to the side of the pool for balance. You will begin to build great stability in your standing leg. When you can do twenty reps with confidence, step away from the side of the pool and balance as you do the exercise. When that gets easy, add resistance blades to regain strength. To make it more challenging, stand on a step as in Photos 9-39A to 9-39E.

Recovering from hip arthroscopy: As soon as you are allowed in the water, you can start this exercise without using any resistance. Focus on squeezing your gluteal muscles each time you reach your leg straight back or back at the angle shown in Photo 9-40B. This is a great exercise for strengthening your gluteal muscles. After six weeks, get your doctor's approval to add resistance pieces as shown in Exercises 9-40A and 9-40B to make the exercise harder for enhanced strength gains.

Recovering from hip implant surgery: Assuming you did Exercise 39, you can skip this one, which was developed primarily for hip arthroscopy patients who need to strengthen their gluteal muscles.

You've made it through the surgery, and you have firmly established our pool program as a source for healing for the rest of your life. Enjoy your time in the water. Build pool time into your weekly schedule from now on. Don't be surprised to learn, as many of our previous patients have, that if you give up the pool, you can easily start slipping down the Negative Spiral of pain and loss of motion. You're working hard for your gains. It's easier to keep them than to have to earn them back again.

11

THE TRANSITION FROM POOL TO LAND

with Ashley White, DPT

"In water my hip doesn't hurt and my exercises feel so easy. Why do I need a land program at all?"

This is the question most frequently asked by patients who have been using the pool program to rehabilitate their hips, and of course the answer is, because you live on land, and also because:

- you may have chlorine-sensitive skin
- some days you're simply stuck at home
- in a pool your ears may be prone to infection
- the pool may be unreasonably far from your home
- your home pool isn't heated in the winter
- you may be incontinent

But your main reason for exercising on land is that your activities of daily living (**ADLs**) take place there, not in buoyancy, but in gravity. When you can perform your ADLs with decreased pain and greater ease of movement, you improve the quality of your daily life. Plus, exercising on land loads weight onto your bones, which provides stimulus to develop healthy bone density and prevent osteoporosis.

When you started reading this book, there may have been many movements you couldn't even imagine doing on land. Yet amazingly, you found that you could tolerate those same movements in a pool because of the comfort and buoyancy of the water. By doing your exercises in the water, you were able to stretch and strengthen your muscles through their normal range of motion, bringing about decreased tightness and pain. Even more important, you were able to do the exercises correctly, because you weren't having to control all your body weight against gravity. Exercising with good form is the only way to create good posture and efficient movement, so congratulate yourself for finding the magic of water to help you through your first steps on your road to recovery.

Had you started on land, you may have felt hip pain and found that the muscles around your hip weren't strong enough to do the exercises you wanted to do. Those weak muscles would have recruited stronger muscles nearby to help you to avoid hip pain, and you could have created bad-habit patterns. For example, you might have overworked your lower back due to your loss of hip motion.

Consider your exercises performed in water to be an incredible stepping-stone to land. You can now move correctly with good form, and you are prepared to tolerate the weight-bearing activities that you do today and every day. As you begin your land exercises, you will gradually get used to gravity's downward pull, which makes your movements different—and harder.

Picture an astronaut on the moon as he jumps, skips, and runs lightly across the surface in his gravity-reduced environment. When he returns to Earth, the movements he performed with such ease become harder. More muscle fibers must fire to do the same tasks. He has to retrain himself to walk, jump, and do other physical activities against Earth's gravity. You'll feel the same change as you move from the pool to land, as if you'd landed back on Earth after being on the moon. Your body will feel heavier, and for a while you'll have to work harder to do the basic skills that were so easy in the pool.

Different laws of physics apply on land. That means different biomechanical rules apply as well—different laws of body movement. For instance, you don't walk the same in the water as you do on land. When you first tried walking in chest-deep water, you probably wobbled at first, having to learn new balance points as you pushed against the water's resistance. You used water's buoyancy to stand tall and walk without bobbing or lurching. As you corrected your gait pattern in the gravity-reduced environment of the water, you strengthened those muscles that are specific to good walking.

With that improved strength, you can make the transition to land. The transition will take time—weeks or even months, depending on the severity of your gait abnormality. When you first try to duplicate your efficient pool alignment on land, you may not be able to maintain an upright posture because your muscles aren't yet strong enough. Yet each time that you reinforce your proper posture in the pool, then try again on land, you get closer to regaining a normal walking pattern. Going back and forth from pool to land, pool to land, allows you to learn from both environments. The water carries most of your weight while you focus on good posture and alignment; at the same time the water's resistance forces strength into the muscles specifically used for walking. Then on land you use the strength, posture, and alignment you developed in the pool to work against gravity.

The same holds true for your other activities of daily living. You took your ADLs for granted before your hip started hurting. Now every curb, ramp, or set of stairs can seem like a major obstacle to negotiate. You can relearn these movements that have become difficult on land by entering the water to reduce or eliminate gravity. In that way your body becomes skilled and strong in the functions necessary for your daily life on land. The result is improved **functionability**, which is the ability to function well within your specific environment. For instance, if you live in a house with seven steps, you need to be able to negotiate those steps without difficulty. You should be able to get safely into bed, the shower, and the bathtub, and in and out of the car and the easy chair. Yet hip pain often limits your ability to perform these basic activities.

Your job is to restore functionability so you can do the things your personal environment requires of you. If you need to be able to perform a specific movement that wasn't offered to you in chapters 9 or 10, create your own pool exercise to generate the skill and strength that will eventually allow you to transition that movement onto land. For example, if it's difficult for you to vacuum your rug, simulate the vacuuming movement in the pool. After many repetitions, you'll be able to do that movement on land.

How to Get In and Out of Your Car

When a sore hip doesn't allow much movement, getting in and out of a car can seem like a major accomplishment. Here's how to make it easy and as pain-free as possible. Note the variations offered if you need extra help.

Getting In

- Open the door.
- Turn your back toward the car seat and sit down, using your hands for control if needed.
- Lift both knees and swing them together into the car in one movement. At the same time, rotate your torso toward the front of the car.
- Sit upright with your back fully against the seat back.
- Variation 1: Use your arms to help lift your legs into the car.
- Variation 2: Hook the foot of your stronger leg behind the ankle of the weaker one to assist the affected leg into the car.

Continued p.204

Getting Out
- Continue to face forward and scoot to the edge of the seat as far as possible.
- Open the door.
- Simultaneously turn your torso and swing both legs to the side of the open door.
- Facing the open door, scoot even closer to the edge of the seat.
- Plant both feet firmly on the ground to prevent any slips or falls as you exit.
- Lean your trunk forward.
- Place your left hand on the doorjamb and your right hand on the door so you can use your upper body strength to assist you in standing.
- Variation 1: Use your arms to assist in moving your legs out of the vehicle.
- Variation 2: Hook the foot of your stronger leg behind the ankle of the weaker one to assist the affected leg out of the car.

Exercise Is Vital

Muscular strength around a damaged joint can take over some of the joint's function. Instead of asking your hip joints to do all the work of supporting your body against gravity, strong muscles—your quadriceps, gluteals, hamstrings, abductors, and others—can do much of that job. If muscles provide a solid support around a hip joint, they take pressure off the weight-bearing surfaces by decreasing friction, swelling, and pain, therefore slowing the deterioration.

Finding Balance

Although symmetry is emphasized in both the pool and land programs, the human body is not actually symmetrical—you probably have one foot or one hand that is slightly larger than the other. Degenerative changes to the body don't happen symmetrically either. Yet your body works symmetrically and your instincts are **bilateral**. You use both feet, both knees, both elbows, and both hips, and if you fall, both hands reach out to break your fall. Therefore your goal is to keep both sides of your body working efficiently. Both hips must be equally strong and limber: you should exercise both hips—the painful one to its maximum tolerance and your healthy hip just enough to keep it strong while the weaker one catches up. Since asymmetry can cause abnormal wear and tear on muscles and joints, you want to maintain balance throughout your body and perform the exercises in this book, all of which promote symmetry.

Which Is Your Dominant Leg?

We all know we're right- or left-handed, but most people don't realize they also have a dominant right or left leg. Professional basketball players, Olympic high jumpers, and other top athletes are well aware that they have a favorite takeoff leg for jumping, and each of us has a preferred leg for movement, whether we know it or not. If your hip problem is your dominant leg, you might find that even a small amount of joint damage can cause severe limitations in your daily function, whereas if the problem hip is your non-dominant leg, you might be able to live with that problem for a longer time.

Think about the last time you rode your bicycle when it was in disrepair. Perhaps the chain was loose and the pedals hesitated at every rotation. Maybe your wheels wobbled because the spokes needed balancing. If you ignored your bike long enough, it might even have made a grinding sound in the bottom bracket where your pedals and crank arm are attached. The bike couldn't operate properly with all those parts malfunctioning, but once you tightened the chain, balanced the spokes of the wheels, and lubricated the bearings in the bottom bracket, you created harmony, stability, and balance. You got a smoother ride.

Your body also needs to be well maintained if you want a smooth ride through your daily activities. Your muscles work in synchronized pairs that need to be balanced. When half of a muscle pair contracts, the opposing one relaxes. The muscle pairs of the hip are the flexors/extensors, abductors/adductors, and internal rotators/external rotators. (See Drawings 2-3 to 2-6 on page 20.) Muscle pairs around a healthy hip retain a specific ratio of strength to each other; around an unhealthy hip, that balance is lost. Most commonly, one-half of a muscle pair becomes tight and restrictive while the other half becomes weak and overstretched.

The typical hip patient has tight adductors and weak abductors, tight flexors and weak extensors, and tight internal rotators and weak external rotators. To correct such imbalances, you need to stretch the tight muscles and strengthen the weak ones. Start by stretching the tight muscles first to increase your range of motion; then strengthen the weak muscles through the newly established range.

Manual Stretches and Resistance Exercises

Every muscle has sensors embedded in the tissues. These sensors, the **muscle spindle** and the Golgi tendon organ, tell the muscles and tendons what to do—when to contract (shorten) or when to relax (lengthen). If a muscle is stretched quickly, the spindle in the belly of the muscle will tell that muscle to contract against the stretch to maintain its usual length; but if a muscle is stretched very slowly with steady, uninterrupted pressure, the spindle stops asking for a contraction and the Golgi tendon organ deep in the tendon starts asking the tissues to relax and lengthen to protect against being torn. The stretching technique discussed on the following pages works with these two sensors to produce positive results. (You learned about the Golgi tendon organ's other function of providing you with position sense on page 74.)

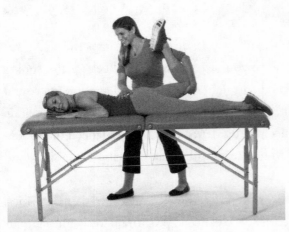
Photo 11-1. Passive, sustained stretch of right hip flexor by therapist.

If your right hip flexor muscles are tight, a physical therapist can have you lie on your stomach as in Photo 11-1 and apply a **passive, sustained stretch** by lifting your right thigh off the table as high as possible and holding it there for thirty seconds. You will feel discomfort at first, but that will subside as the stretch is maintained. As your muscles release, the therapist applies more pressure within your tolerance to constantly challenge your hip flexors to the new, increased range of motion.

HEAL YOUR HIPS

Next, to strengthen the opposite muscle group, the weak hip extensors, you'll perform **repeated contractions** against resistance offered by the therapist. Working through your newly established end-range of motion, push hard and fast ten times against the therapist's hand, and then hold the contraction steady while the therapist counts to five (Photo 11-2). You'll do this several times until the extensors begin to fatigue. Fatigue causes tissue breakdown, then the muscle rebuilds itself, coming back stronger.

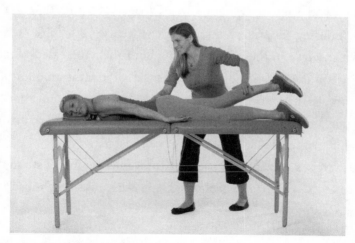

Photo 11-2. Repeated contractions of right extensors with therapist.

The same sustained, passive stretch can be applied to any tight muscles around the hip, and repeated contractions performed to strengthen weak muscles.

Training Muscles in Their Primary Function

Some muscles are primarily movers; others are primarily stabilizers. Your hip flexors and extensors are primarily movers; they move your legs forward and backward. Your external and internal hip rotators are primarily stabilizers; most of the time they work to stabilize your hips. Although your hip abductors and adductors can cause movement, most of the time they, too, stabilize your hips. For instance, your abductors work as movers when you lift your leg to the side, but that's a movement seldom performed in daily life. Rather, the abductors primarily keep your pelvis from collapsing with each step as you walk, run, and go about your day: they are primarily stabilizers.

When you strengthen a muscle, you want to exercise it the way it normally functions. Movers should be strengthened with movement exercise while stabilizers should be strengthened with **isometric** exercise—a contraction of the muscle against a resistance with little or no movement. When you walk, you are exercising the muscles in their correct way: the abductors, adductors, internal rotators, and external rotators stabilize the hips, while the flexors and extensors move the legs forward and backward.

Some pool exercises ask the stabilizers to perform active movement, as in Exercise 35, Lateral Leg Raises (page 163), and Exercise 37, Leg Circles (pages 164 and 165), for a reason. In those specific exercises you're using the water's buoyancy to increase your hip's range of motion. You're also developing equal strength in the muscles throughout their increased range of motion. When you perform a leg circle in the water, you encounter exactly the same amount of resistance through every curve of that circular movement. You can't create similar resistance for the hip on land, so it's important to do that key movement in the water. You will also be working on your stability and balance in that and all the other single-leg standing pool exercises.

Some of the land exercises in chapter 12 use active movement at first to strengthen your abductors, adductors, internal rotators, and external rotators. This is because your muscles are out of balance and require remedial measures.

Turn to chapter 12 to begin your land program and move closer to your goal of regaining a normal gait plus full, symmetrical function in everyday life.

12

A LAND PROGRAM FOR HIP PATIENTS

with Ashley White, DPT

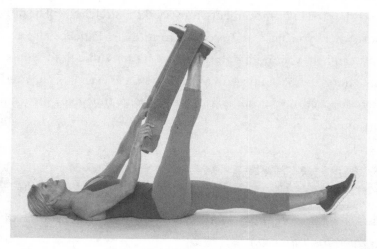

Photo 12-1. Hamstring Stretch.

Exercises 1 through 6 are stretching exercises; Exercises 7 through 26 improve your strength, coordination, balance, and ability to function. If you do them all on a regular basis, you'll feel the difference in your hip and want to make this program a lifelong habit.

Warm-Up Stretches

In all your warm-up stretches, stretch the unaffected hip first so you can focus on good posture and alignment without the distraction of pain. Stretch to a point of slight discomfort, then ease off the stretch just a fraction so the stretch will still be challenging, yet you'll be able to hold it for thirty seconds. While you hold the stretch, breathe deeply and try to relax more deeply with every exhalation. Don't push yourself. A slow stretch held for thirty seconds lets gravity do the work for you. While stretching your healthy hip, pay careful attention to where you feel the stretch so you can compare what you feel to the other side. Then slowly, slowly attempt the stretch on the affected hip, stopping at the point at which you begin to feel pain. Relax just slightly so the pain goes away but you still feel the stretch. Stay there and breathe deeply, monitoring the amount of discomfort you feel. This will lessen over the next weeks, so pay attention. Describe what you feel in a rehab journal, or, if you're in a physical therapy program, report to your therapist the changes you feel.

If your hip is fairly limited in its movements, most of these stretches will be difficult at first. Don't be discouraged! Start where you start, and progress from there. Patience and consistency are what count. Your therapist can help you modify the stretch if it's too difficult for you at first. If you can't easily get down to the floor and back up again, you can perform exercises on your bed.

Establish an exercise space in your home. Choose a specific time to be there and let nothing stop you, short of an earthquake.

Exercise 1. Hamstring Stretch

If you have a back condition, keep one knee bent with your foot on the floor while you raise the other leg.

Lie on your back with a towel or strap around the ball of your foot. Slowly lift your unaffected leg toward the ceiling and straighten your knee until you feel a stretch along the back of your thigh and knee (see Photo 12-1 on page 209). Flex your foot toward your head as shown. Keep your knee as straight as possible. Hold the stretch while you breathe slowly and deeply at least five times. When you feel the muscles relax, first try to straighten the knee more fully, then gently lift your leg higher. Now perform the stretch slowly on your affected leg. Notice any differences between the two legs. Repeat on both sides.

Exercise 2. Knee to Chest Stretch

You may be able to do this exercise one week after surgery, but get your surgeon's approval first. He or she may ask you not to lift your knee so high.

Lie on your back with your legs straight. Keep your head and lower back flat on the floor throughout this stretch. Pull the knee of your unaffected leg toward your chest as in Photo 12-2. Your affected leg remains flat on the floor unless you feel pain, in which case you can bend it slightly. Hold this stretch while you breathe deeply and slowly at least five times. Consciously relax your muscles with every exhalation. Return to the starting position, then perform the stretch slowly on your affected side. As you breathe deeply, you may be surprised to feel your sore hip gain a bit more movement with each breath. Repeat on each side.

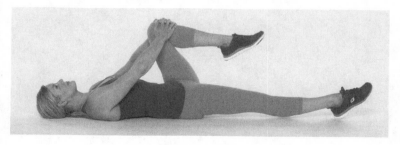

Photo 12-2. Knee to Chest Stretch.

If you have had hip surgery, get your surgeon's approval before doing this exercise.

Lie on your back. Use your hand to pull the knee of your unaffected leg toward your opposite shoulder until you feel a stretch in the buttocks. (See Photo 12-3.) If you feel any pain or pinching in the front of the hip, release the stretch slightly by lowering your knee a bit, but continue pulling the leg across your body. Let your affected leg lie flat on the floor, or you can bend the knee slightly if you feel pain. Hold this stretch while you breathe deeply and slowly at least five times. Consciously relax your muscles with every exhalation. Return to the starting position, then perform the stretch slowly on your affected side. Repeat on each side.

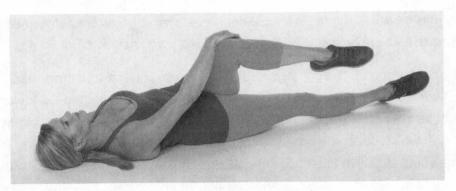

Photo 12-3. Hip Extensor Stretch.

Exercise 4. Iliotibial Band (ITB) Stretch

If you have had hip surgery, get your surgeon's approval before doing this exercise.

Stretching your iliotibial band (ITB) can be difficult, so start gently. Lie on your back with a strap or towel around the foot of your unaffected leg. Lift your leg straight up and then across your midline until you feel a stretch on the outer portion of your hip and down toward your knee. (See Photo 12-4.) Hold this stretch while you breathe deeply and slowly at least five times. As your flexibility improves, you can hold the stretch longer or do it more than once a day. You want to feel a strong pulling stretch but no pain. Now slowly perform this exercise on your affected side. Repeat on each side.

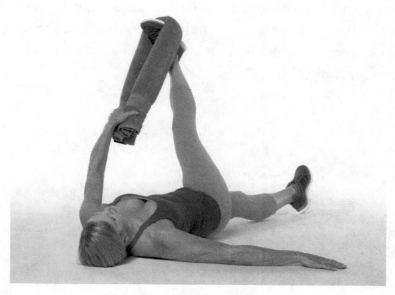

Photo 12-4. Iliotibial Band Stretch.

Exercise 5. Snibbe Stretch

Turn over to lie facedown with your affected hip on a smooth surface such as a wooden floor. Turn your head toward the affected side. Place a small towel under the knee of your affected leg. Keep your hips on the floor as flat as possible while you slide your knee as high as you can without encountering pain. (See Photo 12-5.) Expect to feel a gentle pull and stretch of the muscles but not pain.

This stretch is particularly important for those with FAI or those who have had FAI arthroscopic surgery. This stretch can help you loosen the hip joint capsule, allowing for freer movement. The front of your capsule is probably four times thicker than that of someone who does not have FAI. Thus, you should devote significant time to this stretch. Work up to holding the position for two minutes. Release the stretch and repeat four more times. This means you're doing five repetitions of up to two minutes on your affected hip with a short break as you lower the leg between each stretch. Once you feel better mobility in your affected hip, begin doing this stretch also on your unaffected side, but only one repetition of two minutes.

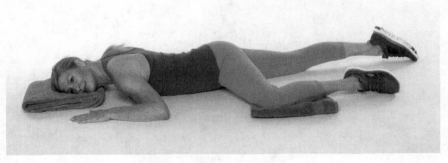

Photo 12-5. Snibbe Stretch.

HEAL YOUR HIPS

Continue to lie facedown with your head turned to the side. Wrap a strap or towel around the foot of your unaffected leg. Use both hands to slowly pull your heel toward your buttocks as in Photo 12-6. Pull until you feel a stretch across the front of your thigh. Be sure your hips do not lift off the ground during the stretch. Hold this stretch while you breathe deeply and slowly at least five times. Next perform the exercise on your affected leg. Repeat on each side.

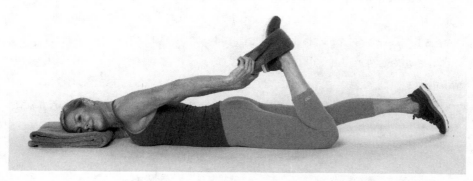

Photo 12-6. Prone Quad Stretch.

Basic Exercises

In the exercises that follow, you'll be asked to perform a specific number of repetitions (reps) of each exercise. Pay attention to what you're feeling. Get to know the strengths and weaknesses of each of the muscle groups so your internal monitoring system will become more developed. That way you'll be able to progress intelligently on your own, or you'll be able to provide your therapist with more valuable information. Do your first set of repetitions with the unaffected hip first; then repeat with your affected hip. Try to duplicate with your affected hip the good movement patterns of your healthy hip. Your goal is to reach equal strength and flexibility in both hips. If you strengthen and stretch one hip, you must also strengthen and stretch the other. Give your healthy hip only a moderate amount of workload to keep it functioning and strong while you work the affected hip to its maximum so it can begin to "catch up" with the healthy hip.

Most people with hip pain have an imbalance in their muscle strength. They usually need to strengthen their extensors and their abductors (see Drawings 2-4 and 2-5 on page 20). These are key muscles in stabilizing the pelvis during walking.

Waking Up Your Hip

You may have increased pain or soreness at some point during the first few weeks, but don't worry. Nothing's going wrong. You're reactivating something that was lying dormant, so don't let the discomfort alarm you. Moving your "rusty" hip is like a bear waking from its long winter nap. It yawns and growls and shows its teeth a little before it gets up to resume its life. Continue with the exercises. As you consistently do the exercises over the weeks and months, you'll see the results. There will be less and less pain and more and more mobility. *If the pain does not decrease after several weeks, discontinue what you are doing and return to your doctor or physical therapist.*

Exercise 7. Prone Hip Extension

Continue to lie facedown with your head turned to the side. Contract your buttocks and abdominal muscles to stabilize your torso. Keep your knees straight and slowly raise your unaffected leg off the floor as in Photo 12-7. Focus on primarily using your buttocks muscles. Hold the leg up for two seconds, then slowly return it to the floor. Do this ten times, and then repeat on the affected side. You can turn your head to the opposite side any time you wish.

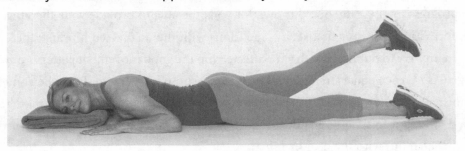

Photo 12-7. Prone Hip Extension.

HEAL YOUR HIPS

Exercise 8. Straight Leg Raise

If you have FAI, have had arthroscopic surgery for FAI, or have hip flexor tendinitis, skip this exercise.

Turn onto your back with the palms of your hands flat on the floor beside your hips. Your unaffected leg is straight and your affected leg is bent with the foot on the floor as in Photo 12-8A. Pull your toes toward you and tighten the quadriceps on your straight leg. Your lower back and both hips stay in contact with the floor throughout this exercise. Keeping your knee straight and your quads tight, slowly lift your straight leg to the level of your bent knee as in Photo 12-8B. Hold the leg up for two seconds, then slowly return it to the floor. Do this ten times; then repeat on the affected side.

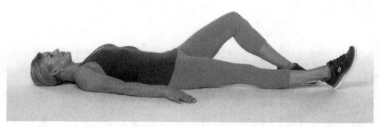

Photo 12-8A. Straight Leg Raise.

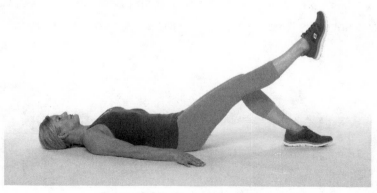

Photo 12-8B. Straight Leg Raise.

Exercise 9. Ball Squeeze with Abdominal Contraction

Lie on your back with a ball or pillow between your knees as in Photo 12-9. Both knees are bent and your feet are on the floor. Allow your back to rest in its natural position on the floor, don't flatten your back to the floor. Tighten your abdominal muscles. Squeeze your knees together and hold for five seconds. Perform ten reps.

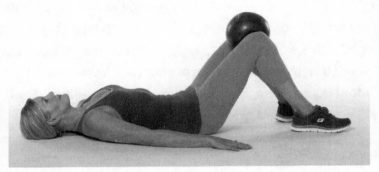

Photo 12-9. Ball Squeeze with Abdominal Contraction.

Exercise 10. Bridge

Remove the ball and continue lying on your back with your knees bent and your feet flat on the floor. See Photo 12-10A. Allow your back to rest in its natural position on the floor as you contract your abdominal muscles. Contract your gluteal muscles, and lift your buttocks off the floor to the position shown in Photo 12-10B. Hold for five seconds before returning to the starting position. Do ten reps.

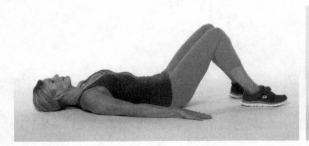

Photo 12-10A. Bridge.

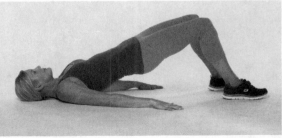

Photo 12-10B. Bridge.

HEAL YOUR HIPS

Exercise 11. Side-Lying Hip Abduction

Lie on your unaffected side with your knee bent to approximately 45 degrees as in Photo 12-11A. Keep your hips and toes pointed straight forward. Lift your affected leg about a foot off the ground. See Photo 12-11B. If you can't raise your leg that high, lift as high as you can. Hold your leg up for two seconds, then slowly lower it to the floor. Do this ten times. If you can turn to lie on your affected side, repeat the exercise with your unaffected leg.

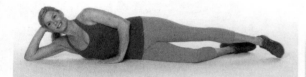

Photo 12-11A. Side-Lying Hip Abduction.

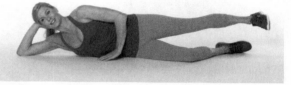

Photo 12-11B. Side-Lying Hip Abduction.

Exercise 12. Clamshell

If you have FAI, have had arthroscopic surgery for FAI, or have hip flexor tendinitis, skip this exercise.

Lie on your side with your affected hip up, one hip directly above the other. Bend your hips to approximately 45 degrees and your knees to 90 degrees as seen in Photo 12-12A. Your feet should be in line with your hips and your shoulders. Keeping your feet in contact with each other, lift your top knee upward as in Photo 12-12B; then slowly return to the starting position. Do this ten times. If you can, turn to lie on your affected side, and repeat with the unaffected side.

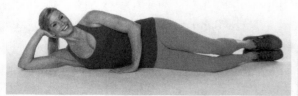

Photo 12-12A. Clamshell.

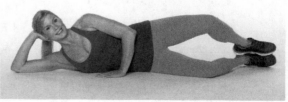

Photo 12-12B. Clamshell.

Assume a balanced position on your hands and knees as in Photo 12-13A. Then lift your unaffected leg out behind you until it is parallel with the floor as in Photo 12-13B. Return to the starting position on your hands and knees. Do ten repetitions on each side.

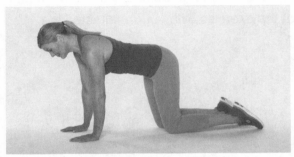

Photo 12-13A. Hip Extension.

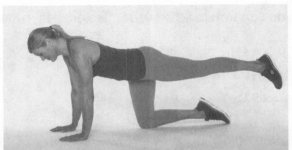

Photo 12-13B. Hip Extension.

Resistance Exercises with Thera-Bands

Chart A. Steps in Thera-Band Progression

Yellow:	One set of ten reps
	Two sets of ten reps
	Three sets of ten reps
Red:	Two sets of ten reps
	Three sets of ten reps
Green:	Two sets of ten reps
	Three sets of ten reps
Blue:	Two sets of ten reps
	Three sets of ten reps

Stretchy latex bands can be used to create resistance and increase your workload. Thera-Bands, as they're called, are six inches wide and come in standard colors that designate their graded resistance. Yellow is the easiest to stretch, then red, green, and blue in increasing order of resistance. Extra resistance makes your muscles work harder, and they will quickly gain strength. You'll perform Exercises 14 through 17 against gradually increasing resistance. You'll want to adjust the position of the band as necessary so you can move through your fullest range of motion without pain. First try the exercises below without a Thera-Band to perfect the execution of the exercise. Then, when you're ready, add the resistance.

As you gain strength each week, you'll progress through the Thera-Bands as shown in Chart A. Move from the yellow to the red Thera-Band only when the exercises become easy and you need more resistance. Use that same criterion moving to green, then blue.

Exercise 14. Hip Extension with Thera-Band

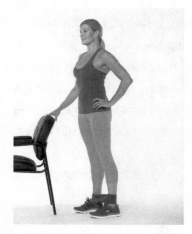

Photo 12-14A. Hip Extension with Thera-Band.

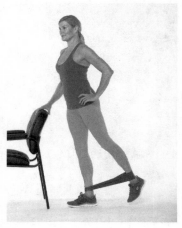

Photo 12-14B. Hip Extension with Thera-Band.

Tie the ends of the Thera-Band together to create a loop and circle it around both your lower legs. Place one or both of your hands on a chair or table for support as in Photo 12-14A. Engage your buttocks and abdominal muscles as you reach your unaffected leg straight backward as shown in Photo 12-14B. Keep your knees straight through the entire exercise. Adjust your position closer to or farther away from the chair as necessary. If you stand too close, there won't be any resistance for the beginning of the exercise. If you stand too far away, you won't be able to pull your leg backward through the full range of motion. This position may change over a period of weeks; as you gain strength, you'll be able to pull harder against the band.

Keep your abdominals engaged throughout this exercise. Don't arch your back as you reach your leg behind you. The goal of this exercise is to work the buttocks muscles, not the muscles in your lower back.

When you finish one set of ten reps, perform a set with your affected leg. Switch back and forth until you've completed your sets and reps.

Do the number of sets and reps you've mastered. See Chart A on page 220.

Exercise 15. Hip Abduction with Thera-Band

Stand with your side to the chair so that your unaffected leg is away from the chair. Both feet are inside the loop of the Thera-Band as in Photo 12-15A. Place your hand on the chair for support, or place both hands on a table if you feel the need. Keep your knee straight and reach your leg to the side as far as you can as shown in Photo 12-15B. Don't let your leg move forward; keep it moving strictly to your side in order to target the proper muscles. Maintain your erect posture; don't lean so you can reach the leg farther to the side. Adjust your position to the chair depending on what you feel. If it's too easy, move away from the chair. If it's too hard, move closer. Just make sure that you have some degree of tension in the band throughout the movement. Complete your first set of ten, then repeat with your affected leg.

Do the number of sets and reps you've mastered. See Chart A on page 220.

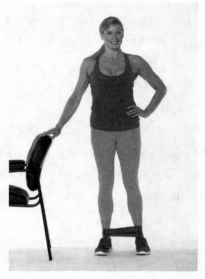

Photo 12-15A.
Hip Abduction with Thera-Band.

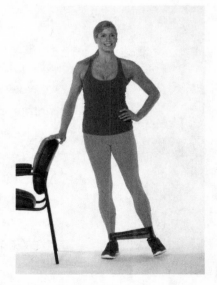

Photo 12-15B.
Hip Abduction with Thera-Band.

HEAL YOUR HIPS

Exercise 16. Hip External Rotation with Thera-Band

Sit on a table or chair that is high enough that your feet won't touch the ground. The backs of your knees should touch the edge of the table. Place the foot of your unaffected leg inside the Thera-Band as shown in Photo 12-16A. Use your hands to brace yourself as you pull against the Thera-Band so that your foot moves inward and your knee and hip rotate outward (external rotation), as shown in Photo 12-16B. Don't let your thigh move across the table; only your lower leg should be moving. Adjust your position to the table leg depending on what you feel. If it's too easy, move away from where the Thera-Band is attached. If it's too hard, move closer. Just make sure that you have some degree of tension in the band throughout the movement. Complete your first set of ten; then repeat with your affected leg.

Do the number of sets and reps you've mastered. See Chart A on page 220.

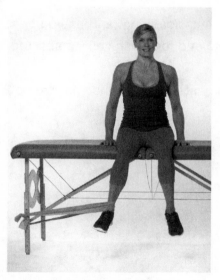

Photo 12-16A. Hip External
Rotation with Thera-Band.

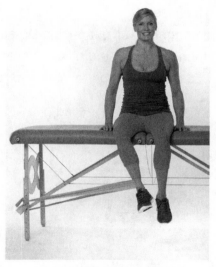

Photo 12-16B. Hip External
Rotation with Thera-Band.

If you've had hip implant surgery, get your surgeon's approval before doing this exercise.

Continue to sit on the table or chair where your feet don't touch the ground. Move the Thera-Band to the opposite leg of the table or chair to perform internal rotation. Use your hands to brace yourself as you pull against the Thera-Band so that your foot moves outward and your knee and hip rotate inward (internal rotation), as shown in Photo 12-17B. Don't let your thigh move across the table; only your lower leg should be moving. Adjust your position to the table leg depending on what you feel. If it's too easy, move away from where the Thera-Band is attached. If it's too hard, move closer. Just make sure that you have some degree of tension in the band throughout the movement.

This exercise may feel a bit awkward if you are not in tune with isolating these smaller muscles during daily activities. However, the more you do this exercise the more you will feel the correct muscles firing, and as you become stronger, it will get easier. Do all of your sets and reps with your unaffected leg, then repeat on the affected side.

Do the number of sets and reps you've mastered. See Chart A on page 220.

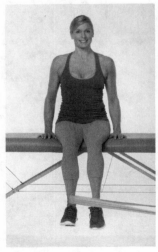

Photo 12-17A.
Hip Internal Rotation with Thera-Band.

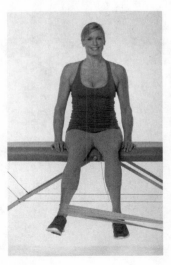

Photo 12-17B.
Hip Internal Rotation with Thera-Band.

Stability Ball Exercises

These exercises don't work an isolated muscle group such as you did in many of the previous exercises. You aren't working just your gluteals, hip flexors, or hamstrings. Instead, in Exercises 18 through 20, you are engaging the core and using your muscles **synchronistically**; that is, you are coordinating the work of various muscles to create smooth, efficient movement.

Together, your nerves and muscles work to produce movements. Your brain sends signals down your nerves to your muscles about where, when, and how fast to move. It is a complex process. Over time, nerve pathways are reinforced, and muscle movement patterns are learned and stored in your memory. You have probably heard people discuss what is called "muscle memory." This is why you remember how to walk up and down steps and automatically know how to adjust your movements for taller or shorter steps. But such automatic muscle movement patterns are affected when nerves or muscles are damaged or injured. When your hip joint is painful and you go through the Negative Spiral, as on page 22, your muscles and nerves become part of your hip dysfunction. This means that besides regaining the range of motion of your hip and increasing the strength in your muscles that surround the hip, you need to retrain your nerves and muscles. That's called **neuromuscular reeducation**. When the nerve signals are "retrained" and appropriate muscle movements are repeated, movement patterns become automatic again. The end goal is to regain your efficient patterns of motion.

As you do the exercises in this section, be aware that you are getting back the **synchronicity** of the working muscles. You are teaching those muscles to fire correctly and improving your muscle-firing pattern—muscle A fires first, then muscle B, then C. When you train the muscles around both your hips to fire in the same correct pattern, your body regains symmetry for improved function.

These three exercises begin with a basic Bridge on the stability ball as in Exercise 18. For Exercises

19 and 20, start in the same position as shown in Photo 12-18B and continue to the more advanced positions that follow. If Exercises 19 and 20 prove too difficult for you, make it your goal to perform two to three sets of ten repetitions of the basic Bridge, Exercise 18.

Exercise 18. Bridge on Ball

Lie on your back on the floor and place a stability ball under your ankles as shown in Photo 12-18A. Flatten your back and squeeze your buttocks. Then lift your buttocks as high as you comfortably can and hold for five seconds as in Photo 12-18B. Do this ten times.

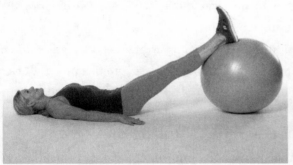
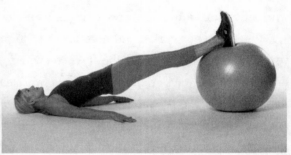

Photo 12-18A. Bridge on Ball.   Photo 12-18B. Bridge on Ball.

Exercise 19. Bridge on Ball with Leg Lift

Continue lying on the floor with a fitness ball under your ankles. Flatten your back and squeeze your buttocks. Lift your buttocks off the floor as shown in Photo 12-18B. Continue holding this position as you do the next movement. Tighten all of the muscles in your unaffected leg. It will be stabilizing you as you lift your affected leg toward the ceiling (Photo 12-19) and then lower it back to the ball. You may feel wobbly, so use your arms for control. Next let your affected leg do the stabilizing and lift your unaffected leg. Lower your unaffected leg to the ball and lower your buttocks to the floor. Do ten repetitions, lifting first your

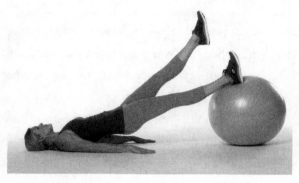

Photo 12-19. Bridge on Ball with Leg Lift.

affected and then your unaffected leg each time you lift up into the bridge. As you are learning this exercise, you can lower your hips to the floor after each left-right leg raise. As you progress, try to hold your hips up throughout your entire series of reps.

Exercise 20. Bridge on Ball with Hamstring Curl

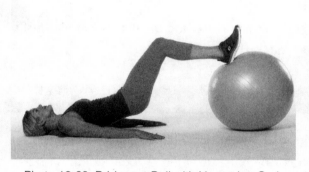

Photo 12-20. Bridge on Ball with Hamstring Curl.

Continue lying on the floor with your ankles on the ball as shown in Photo 12-18A. Flatten your back, then engage your buttocks muscles as you lift your hips up to the basic Bridge position shown in Photo 12-18B. Use your arms for stability. Keeping your heels in contact with the ball, bend your knees as you roll the ball closer to your body. See Photo 12-20. Hold for five seconds, then straighten your legs out to the starting position. As you first try this exercise, you can lower your buttocks to the starting position between reps. But as you get stronger, keep your hips up the entire time while you do your repetitions. Aim for ten reps, but if that's too hard, start with five reps and add one each session until you reach ten.

Balance Exercises

Throughout your daily activities, even when you're not thinking about it, your body is working to maintain your balance. You may be standing in line at the bank and notice that you sway slightly forward and backward as you maintain your upright stance. That balance mechanism is largely an automatic reflex that often employs your ankles and your hips. The hip is a part of the **pelvic girdle**, which is one of the key areas of your body that creates your stability and balance. So you can imagine if your hip is painful or if you have had hip surgery, it may be more difficult for you to maintain your balance. When you move, your brain will alter the firing of the muscles to try to avoid your problematic hip. This happens even without your being aware of it, and it potentially throws off your balance. It can make activities more difficult, such as reaching down to pick up a dog's ball or turning around quickly when someone calls your name.

With practice, anyone can achieve better balance. It just takes consistency and dedication to doing the exercises. As your hip regains its strength and mobility, your brain no longer detours the balancing reflexes elsewhere. And as your legs get stronger and your ankles more flexible, these improvements will allow you to catch yourself even if you do trip.

You can do Exercises 21 through 23 almost anytime, anywhere, and as often as you like. Just be sure to have something solid within arm's reach as you work on your balance.

Exercise 21. Single Leg Balance

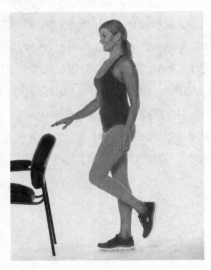

Photo 12-21. Single Leg Balance.

Stand in front of a chair, counter, or solid surface that you can hold for balance. Find a focal point, stand erect, and engage your abdominals and buttocks. Slowly let go of the chair. Once you feel stable, lift your affected leg just slightly, which will force you to balance on the unaffected leg as shown in Photo 12-21. Stand for fifteen seconds or until you lose your balance and need to hold on to the counter or solid surface. Perform the same exercise while standing on the affected leg. Repeat on each side. Each day that you do this exercise, try to add at least one second to your balancing time. Make thirty seconds your goal and work your way up to that.

HEAL YOUR HIPS

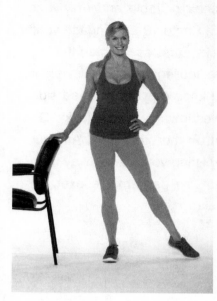

Photo 12-22. Clocks with Single Leg Balance, leg to person's nine o'clock.

Stand erect in front of a mirror. Have a chair nearby so you can rest your hand on it in case you lose your balance. Maintain good posture and tighten your abdominals. Stand only on your unaffected leg with the knee slightly bent. Imagine that you are standing in the center of a large clock's face and twelve o'clock is straight ahead of you. In this exercise, you will reach your affected leg as far as you can toward twelve o'clock without losing your balance. If your affected leg is your left one, as shown in Photo 12-22, you will touch your toe at twelve, nine, and six o'clock. If your affected leg is your right one, touch your toe at twelve, three, and six o'clock. Watch yourself in the mirror so you don't allow your standing knee to move from side to side. It should be directly above your standing foot. Each time you touch three points on the clock's face is one rep. Do ten reps.

If keeping your balance is challenging, you may be slightly uncomfortable at first when you are moving from one position to the next. But as your muscles become reeducated on how to support you through these changing postures, it will become easier. In fact, if you do this exercise often enough, you'll soon want to increase your reps as well as take your hand off the chair for an added challenge.

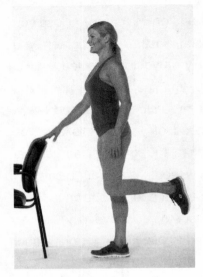

Stand in front of a chair or table and rest your hand on it as shown in Photo 12-23. Engage your abdominal and buttocks muscles. Tighten the leg muscles of your unaffected leg and put your weight on that leg. Bend the knee on your affected side so that your heel moves toward your buttocks. Do ten reps, then repeat on the other side. As your balance improves, try lifting your hand away from the chair so that you can perform the exercise without losing your balance.

Photo 12-23.
Standing Hamstring Curl.

Functional Exercises

Functional exercises literally recreate the exact motions that you do day in and day out. They simultaneously use multiple muscle groups and joints, which improves your muscular endurance, overall strength, coordination, balance, posture, and agility. These functional exercises simulate common movements you do every day, thereby training your muscles to work together by firing in the correct sequence.

While training on machines isolates muscle groups to strengthen them, it doesn't teach the muscle groups you're isolating to move in coordination with one another. That's what functional exercises do. Each time you precisely perform these exercises, you are retraining your muscles to follow the correct muscle-firing patterns. That will mean smoother, more efficient movements. So do each repetition of Exercises 24 and 25 with awareness of how you are moving. Are you shifting your weight back onto your heels as you should? Are you engaging your core muscles and gluteals as you begin to move? Using good form and being mindful as you move is important, not just doing the exercises. That's the key to getting the most out of these Functional Exercises.

Exercise 24. Sit to Stand

Stand with your back to a sturdy chair that has arms as shown in Photo 12-24A. Your feet are shoulder width apart. Engage your core muscles as you reach your arms behind you toward the arms of the chair. Keep your feet flat on the floor while pushing your weight into your heels. Your weight should be evenly distributed between both legs. Squat as if you are going to sit down as shown in Photo 12-24B. If you are unsure of your balance, place your hands on the armrests for support. Lightly touch your buttocks to the seat of the chair without sitting down, then stand up to the starting position. Use your gluteal muscles to initiate the standing motion. That means you will squeeze your buttocks muscles just before you rise and keep your attention on using them throughout the exercise. Keep your chest up and look at a focal point ahead of you as you move from standing to sitting to standing again. Do ten repetitions.

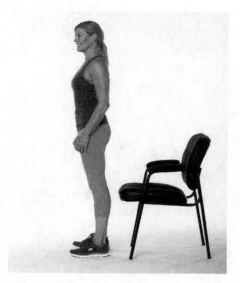
Photo 12-24A. Sit to Stand.

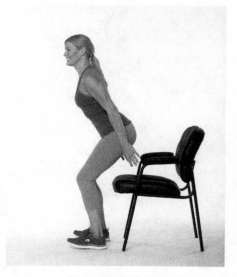
Photo 12-24B. Sit to Stand.

Place the foot of your unaffected leg into the center of a step or block as in Photo 12-25A. That foot will remain in the same position throughout this exercise. In fact, only that one foot will touch the step until you switch sides. Find a focal point in front of you, and keep your eyes locked on that spot to help with balance. Engage your core and buttocks muscles as you begin. Without touching the step with your other foot, lift up over the step (Photo 12-25B), and touch down on the opposite side of the step as in Photo 12-25C. Next, step up and back to the starting position—again, without letting your affected leg touch the step. Your unaffected leg is carrying your weight as you step over and back, yet your affected leg has to touch down, stabilize, and push off on each step. Do ten reps standing on your unaffected leg and then repeat on your affected leg.

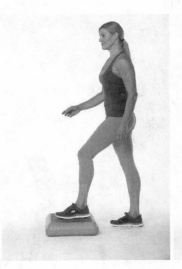
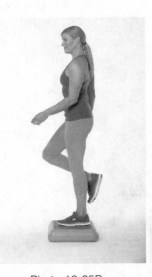
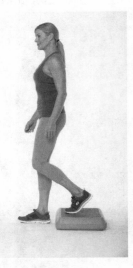

Photo 12-25A.   Photo 12-25B.   Photo 12-25C.

Step Over and Back.

Weight Training

If you had simply gone to the gym and started using the weight-training equipment right away, you might have done yourself harm. You could have easily overloaded your muscles, tendons, or other soft tissues by asking them to do more than they're capable of, and caused more pain, more tightness, and less mobility. It's necessary to start slowly and increase the workload very gradually over time in order to assure yourself of constant gains without major flare-ups or setbacks. By the time you've worked your way to the blue Thera-Band (see chart A on page 220), you will have developed new strength in your hip and will be functioning better in your daily life.

It may be time to start using weight-training machines that create an ever-increasing workload for the muscles. If you're ready to start this kind of training, a trainer or therapist can show you the new equipment. The weight room offers you a variety of exercises that continue to strengthen all the muscles you've been working. Remember that your goal is to help your weak hip catch up with the healthy hip. Thus you'll challenge the weaker one to its maximum while you let the stronger one work at a more moderate level.

If you don't have an affinity for weight training machines, or don't like the idea of training in a gym or health club, you can continue doing all the exercises in this chapter at home. Whatever you decide, know that these exercises are now part of your life.

13

HIP ARTHROSCOPY

with Jason Snibbe, MD

*W*elcome to the chapter about one of the most exciting parts of hip surgery, hip arthroscopy. Our first book told you how I used arthroscopy to try to stop the degeneration of your hip before you would need implant surgery. In those early days, we cleaned out debris from your hip, often a torn labrum. Then in 2003, the term impingement was coined, and we learned that something inside the hip was mechanically tearing the labrum. Since it was a mechanical problem, we could address it with orthopedic surgery. Swiss surgeons used an open procedure to remove the impingement. Then American pioneers began doing the same work arthroscopically.

I was an early believer in hip arthroscopy, so I wrote papers and chapters in books and I spoke at surgical meetings. The hip surgeons were doing implants and wanted nothing to do with the arthroscope. The arthroscopy surgeons who did knees, shoulders, and ankles wanted nothing to do with the hip. To find an audience of surgeons who would be interested in this was difficult for me in the beginning.

In 1994, the former great NBA center Wilt Chamberlain came to me for hip arthroscopy. He understood the concept of trying to solve his hip problem before it needed implant surgery. He told me that water exercises with Lynda Huey would be an important part of his preparation and recovery. Through Lynda's work with Wilt, he recognized the importance of pool therapy before and after surgery. As with all things Wilt touched, both hip arthroscopy and pool therapy gained credibility.

Today, doctors are flocking to courses where they can learn arthroscopic hip surgery. So it is very gratifying to have been a part of envisioning and anticipating the future as a pioneer in hip arthroscopy. I'm happy to say that is has become the fastest growing part of sports medicine.

With great pleasure, Lynda and I have invited hip arthroscopist Jason Snibbe, MD, to join us in this chapter. He is at the forefront of helping to advance what we can do through the arthroscope as we diagnose and treat the hip.

—Robert Klapper, MD

Arthros in Greek means "joint," and *scope* means "to see inside." During hip arthroscopy we make a tiny puncture site and insert a pencil-sized optical device into the hip joint. A miniature television camera attached to the arthroscope allows us to view the interior of the joint on a large video monitor.

Before arthroscopic procedures became available on the hip joint, traumatic open procedures were necessary to operate inside the joint. Those open procedures meant cutting through the skin and the underlying tissues and dislocating the joint. But now, using the tiny instruments that let us work through a small puncture site, we can easily get past those same structures: the skin, the muscles, the **subcutaneous** tissues, the subcutaneous fat, the ligaments, and the joint capsule. Techniques and instruments have evolved so surgeons can perform hip arthroscopic surgery with hardly any tissue damage from the instruments.

In the pioneering days of arthroscopic hip surgery, we put the scope inside the hip joint for different reasons than we do today. In the 1990s, we intended to "clean out" the hip joint by taking out structures we considered problematic. Today we use the procedure as hip preservation surgery. Where we used to **debride** (trim out) a torn labrum, now we repair or reconstruct that vital structure. Where we used to see extra bone and ignore it, now we understand the impingement, and we sculpt away that extra bone to create more clearance in the joint. This has been a true game changer in hip preservation. In effect, the identification of femoroacetabular impingement (FAI) created a new subcategory of hip diagnoses, most of which could be solved arthroscopically rather than with a larger open procedure.

In 2007, surgical tool companies realized hip arthroscopy was here to stay, and they developed longer, curved instruments to navigate around the large ball of the femoral head, which was blocking our view of the socket. They created surgical anchors that could be passed into the hip and hold grafts in place. These advances allow us to do new, highly-skilled work with miniature tools inside the joint. Additionally, we can correct nearby structures outside the joint capsule that are damaged: a torn gluteus medius tendon, chronic trochanteric bursitis, a snapping hip tendon, or even a hamstring tendon that needs reattaching to the base of the pelvis.

Temporary or Permanent Solutions

Some conditions can be partially or fully resolved with arthroscopy. They are:

• Femoroacetabular Impingement (FAI)
• Torn labrum

- Loose bodies or fragments in the joint
- Synovitis

Femoroacetabular Impingement (FAI)

This is the primary reason people today require hip arthroscopy. There are three types of FAI: pincer, cam, and a combination of the two. About 99 percent of the time, the patients who come to us with FAI and pain also have a torn labrum. The bony prominences impact against each other and often tear the labrum and lead to osteoarthritis. The discovery of FAI is what created the concept of hip preservation. We can now resculpt the bones and eliminate the bony impingement, and that may save many hips from needing implant surgery in the future. (Chapter 5 on page 73 gives a full explanation of FAI.)

Besides improving our skill at salvaging hips, we are continually fine-tuning our criteria for who will do well as a candidate for hip arthroscopy, and who should not have this surgery.

Your Other Hip at Risk

FAI is typically bilateral, so when we operate on one hip, we know that your other hip is at risk for labral damage and needing the same surgery. We want to prevent the other hip from getting injured by educating you on the things that are good or bad to do. Stay away from deep squats and deep flexion exercises—anything that bends your hip more than 90 degrees. If you participate in a sport that requires these movements, do them *only* during competition; don't do dozens of repetitions in training that can injure your hip. Begin doing traction on your non-operative hips—a lot of people who have FAI love it! See pages 170 to 171 for deep-water traction, called Hip Distraction, which you can do for yourself at the end of your pool sessions.

—Jason Snibbe, MD

Torn Labrum

The labrum is a rim of fibrocartilage that runs completely around the acetabulum (the socket side of the hip joint), effectively deepening the socket and increasing the "capture" of the socket onto the ball. In the early 2000s, a torn labrum was removed, just as an entire torn meniscus in the knee was removed in the 1970s. But in the 1980s, when knee arthroscopy became commonplace, doctors recognized how important it was to save as much of the meniscus as possible. Similarly today, doctors understand the role of the labrum of the hip and want to retain it at all costs. We now know its main function is to provide the seal that holds in the joint fluid, keeping the hip lubricated. That seal also maintains the negative pressure within the hip joint, which we believe is a good environment for the cartilage. It also helps create stability in the joint and acts as a protective cushion between the edge of the acetabulum (socket) and the constantly moving femoral head (ball). Thus we no longer "clean out" a torn labrum as we used to. Instead, we want to repair or reconstruct it.

Loose Bodies

Loose bodies are benign fragments inside the joint, usually made of cartilage or bone. They are commonplace in the FAI setting. In the past, this was the classic reason for hip arthroscopy, but we no longer do many loose-body retrievals except when combined with FAI surgery.

Synovitis

When the synovial lining (synovium) of the hip joint is inflamed, that's synovitis. Trimming out portions of the synovium is an intrinsic part of hip arthroscopy. It happens at each step of the procedure. During hip arthroscopy, we frequently see bright red synovium. We know those tissues are inflamed, so we do a **synovectomy**, a removal of portions of the synovial lining. We use a heating device to **cauterize** it until the discolored tissue is gone. Removing the inflamed tissue reduces the pain. Sometimes we perform a synovectomy in cases where the diagnosis is not clear from the history, physical, or MRI studies, and we need tissue to look at under the microscope to help in making the diagnosis in order to treat the patient correctly.

Success Stories by Dr. Snibbe

A 6'9", 350-pound high school football player from Seattle was recruited on a full scholarship to a Division I college in Los Angeles. Both his hips had been so tight in high school that he couldn't lower himself into a three-point stance on the offensive line. His coaches let him line up in a modified stance because he was the biggest player around and able to get his job done in spite of improper form. However, once in Los Angeles, the high-level coaches insisted on the traditional three-point stance. They told him that he had to get his butt down where it belonged and stay low so that when he was playing opposite other Division I players, they wouldn't knock him right over. He forced himself down into the stance but had so much pain in his hips that he could no longer practice.

He had two incredibly large cam impingements. We took him to surgery and removed a huge cam off one hip; then we did the other hip a month later. The cam impingements will never grow back. The surgery was hard to do. We had to be creative about making the table long enough for his height and also maintaining the ability to provide traction during the surgery.

Six weeks after the surgery, he said he could move his hips better than ever before in his entire life. He was able to get deep into a squat and down into the classic form of a three-point stance. Three months after the surgery, he was doing drills with limited contact. At five months, he was practicing with the team, and at six months, he was playing football with full contact. Now he's a starting offensive lineman at a Division I school and is playing the best football of his life.

That surgery changed the destiny of this young man's life. He can now have a full college career and possibly become an NFL lineman where he may be able to have a successful career. If this surgery hadn't been available, he would have had to live with the hip pain and dysfunction or end up with hip implant surgery at a young age.

An orthopedic surgeon in Orange County had a pincer impingement that had damaged his labrum. As a serious skier and cyclist, he wanted to have a highly functioning hip. During his surgery, I saw that his labrum was completely calcified. That can happen if the pincer impingement is significant enough that it bangs against the labrum repeatedly. To protect itself, the labrum calcifies—it basically becomes bone. I knew I had to reconstruct the labrum. First, I reduced the pincer impingement. Then I built him a new labrum. I made an incision on his thigh and took a piece of his iliotibial band. I rolled it up like a cigar to become his new labrum. I stitched the tissue to hold it together in its new shape, then fastened it to the bone so he would have a new, functioning labrum. Three months after his surgery, he could ski and bike without pain.

Let's emphasize that it wasn't just the arthroscopic surgery that helped these patients get better; it was the surgery in partnership with the pool and land exercise programs. You can have the best operation in the world, but if you don't rehab it correctly, you won't get a great result—and water therapy is *key* in the rehab process.

Are You a Candidate for Hip Arthroscopy?

You need to get an official diagnosis to learn if you have an impingement. If you have FAI, is it pincer, cam, or both? Is there also a labral tear? Is it combined with ostheoarthritis?

Unbelievably, it takes an average of six to seven months before a patient with FAI is properly diagnosed. He or she may have been referred from one doctor to another. One might say it's just hip flexor pain or some irritation in the joint. Another might say it's a hernia. Yet another might tell you that your hip isn't so bad; maybe it's your back. Virtually all doctors can see osteoarthritis on an X-ray. But not all are schooled in FAI and labral tears. They may tell you to do some physical therapy and you'll be fine. But if you have a bony impingement, that won't change. That's why you want to know for sure whether you have FAI or not.

When I consider which of my patients makes an ideal candidate for hip arthroscopy, these are the things I consider:

- Do you have FAI with a painful labral tear? This is the most common indication for hip arthroscopy, but if you have too much underlying arthritis, that would be a reason not to do the surgery. Your X-ray may look normal without any arthritis, but your MRI may show more significant degeneration of the joint than was seen on the X-ray, which would make you not a great candidate.
- Have you diligently tried the pool and land programs for at least three months and not found relief from your symptoms? Before we consider any surgery, no matter how minimally invasive it may be, we want to see if it's possible for you to regain strength, flexibility, and function through exercise. If you say you made an honest effort and failed, you may be a candidate.
- How long have you been having symptoms? If you have been having hip pain or dysfunction for six months to a year, we are likely to consider surgery. We don't act quickly; we want you to try to rehab it conservatively first.

- What are the physical demands of your life? If you have FAI and a labral tear, but love to swim freestyle and can do that without any pain, we would leave you alone. But if you say you can't swim well and you're having trouble doing all your favorite activities, then we will want to operate on your hip to allow you to return to your active lifestyle.
- Thirty percent of the world's population has FAI and labral tears of which they are unaware. If your labrum is torn but you're asymptomatic, we wouldn't operate on it. You may have a diagnosis of FAI and a labral tear, but if you're satisfied with your ability to meet the physical demands of your life and if you're not having a significant amount of pain, we would leave you alone.

Everyone wants to avoid the bigger total hip surgery, but not everyone is a candidate for hip arthroscopy. There are three reasons you would *not* be a candidate:

1. If you have arthritic pain that causes limping or if you experience aching in your hip at night. Osteoarthritis is not a reason for hip arthroscopy.
2. If one hip is significantly stiffer than the other. Most people have FAI and limited range of motion on both sides due to the FAI. But when you notice that one hip is significantly stiffer and has lost a significant amount of motion compared to the other side, that's a sign that it's not just FAI, but rather the progression of osteoarthritis.
3. If your MRI shows swelling in the bone, that's an indication of arthritis. When the cartilage is worn away, you get pressure on the bone and that creates swelling in the ball and in the socket, which creates pain and discomfort. It's a clue that the arthritis is significant. That's what causes the aching in the night and the chronic bone pain in the hip. This pain cannot be treated through arthroscopy.

If you fit into one of those three categories, your surgeon may be telling you that you need hip implant surgery. It's always wise to get a second opinion—another doctor may suggest that you first pursue other conservative treatment. But if you eventually do build toward a decision to have hip implant surgery, we'll guide you through it in the next chapter.

Hip Arthroscopic Surgery

If you are a good candidate for hip arthroscopy and have found a surgeon, you'll want to ask him or her what to expect throughout your day in the hospital or surgical center.

For now let us be your guide. On the day of surgery you'll pass through admissions and pre-op and be taken into the operating room (OR) by the nurses and the anesthesiologist. You have probably decided which kind of anesthesia to use—a nerve block, an epidural, a spinal, or a general, and your doctor will confirm your choice with the anesthesiologist, who then administers it. Then you'll be given intravenous (IV) antibiotics to guard against infection. The leg that is to be scoped is treated with an antiseptic solution and draped so that the area of the hip joint and the leg involved is exposed.

Positioning the Patient on the Traction Table

We use a traction table and we generously pad the feet and the post between the patient's legs to protect them during traction. These preparations protect the skin from pressure sores, bruising, or tears in the skin on the top of the foot and around the ankle where the foot goes into the boot. We pad the post between the patient's legs to protect the crotch area against the pressure of traction. We have learned that traction can be placed on a hip for a maximum of two hours before risking nerve problems for the patient.

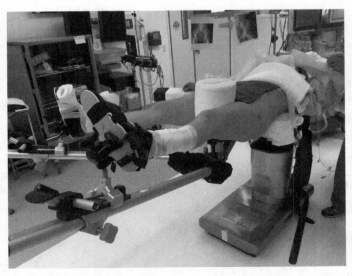

Photo 13-1. The patient's foot is strapped into a boot on the traction table. Dr. Snibbe marks the surgical site to show that's the leg for the operation. Counter-traction is applied to the opposite leg.

Surgery

Let's assume that the patient has a combination of pincer and cam impingement. Our first step is done very carefully and precisely; in fact, most surgeons use X-ray to help guide them. We put a hollow needle inside the hip joint, and once it is inside, air from the outside flows into the hip and releases the negative pressure. That allows us to apply traction to the hip with less force—to separate the ball from the socket so we have room in which to operate. We create two puncture sites on the side of the hip and insert **cannulas**, which are hollow tubes that allow instruments to pass through muscles into the joint without damage. The cannulas provide stable entryways as the surgeon moves instruments in and out of the two openings.

The hip joint capsule is much thicker than other joint capsules in the body. That extra thickness plus the traction pulling tightly on the leg makes it difficult for us to maneuver the instruments around in the joint unless we cut away some of the capsule to gain entry and elbow room, so to speak. We make slices in the capsule in strategic lines that allow us to angle the instruments back and forth inside the hip.

When we first get inside the joint, we become oriented by looking around, doing what we call a diagnostic arthroscopy. We locate the labral tear and the articular cartilage; we look for loose bodies; we look at the labrum in the front of the hip and the labrum at the back of the hip. We look at the **ligamentum teres**, the ligament that connects the femoral head to the acetabulum. People who do extreme movements with their hips such as dancers or gymnasts are predisposed to injuring or tearing this ligament. We often see synovitis on the ligamentum teres, which we think is a source of pain in the hip, so we carefully cauterize it off without harming the ligament. If the ligament is frayed or slightly damaged, we'll trim out frayed portions.

Once we have oriented ourselves to the anatomy, we move our instruments to the bone above the labrum to look for a pincer impingement. If the patient has a true pincer, we peel off the labrum and **burr down** the extra bone to make the outer edge of the acetabulum the correct size, then we reattach the labrum. (See Drawing 13-1 on page 244.) If there isn't a pincer, we simply roughen up the bone to make it bleed so that the labrum will heal to it.

Then we repair the labrum, saving as much of it as possible and reattaching it to the bone. The labrum is a triangular shape, not a round tube, so we don't want to put sutures around it and change its shape. We put the stitches through the meaty part of the labrum to maintain its true anatomical shape, then anchor it to the bone with small, dissolvable plastic devices. We wedge these devices into pre-drilled holes in the bone and pound them down with a miniature hammer. The labrum almost never re-tears after it has been surgically repaired as long as the impingement is fully removed. Some surgeons use X-ray to check that enough bone has been removed in both the pincer and cam defects.

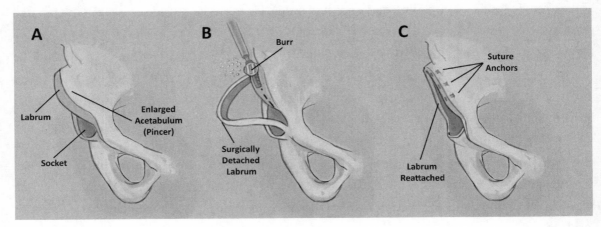

Drawing 13-1.

A. Pincer with enlarged acetabular bone.
B. Labrum is detached during arthroscopic surgery so acetabular bone can be filed down with a surgical burr, removing the pincer.
C. Labrum is reattached with suture anchors to a less prominent bony edge of the socket.

In most cases, there is enough labrum present to repair. But if you have a bad pincer that has done extreme damage to your labrum, it can be so beat up that it's almost gone. If your own labrum is damaged beyond repair, we will need to reconstruct it. We use either cadaver tissue or a small piece of your iliotibial band along the side of your thigh. The general opinion today is to use your own tissue to reconstruct the labrum because we sense that the healing rate to the bone is better.

Whatever tissue we choose to replace your labrum, the first thing we have to do is figure out how long it needs to be. We have a measuring tool inside the joint to measure how long your new labrum should be. We add a little to that to make sure it isn't too short, then we cut the graft, prepare it, and slide it into the hip. We use the same technique of attaching the replacement tissue to the bone as we did in repairing your own labrum: we place stitches through it and anchor it to the bone in the same way.

HEAL YOUR HIPS

We resolve the problems with the pincer and the labrum inside the central compartment of the ball and socket. As soon as we've completed that work, we release the traction on the hip. The ball returns to its normal position inside the socket. You can expect traction to be applied for only forty-five to fifty minutes if your surgeon is experienced. Next we move the camera and instruments to what's called the peripheral compartment to evaluate the cam. We have to cut a little more of the capsule so we can locate the cam formation and burr it down to remove it.

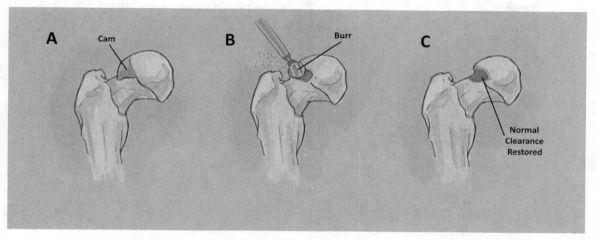

Drawing 13-2. Cam removal surgery can also involve labral repair if needed.

A. Cam with prominent bony bump on the femoral neck.
B. Bone spur is filed down with a surgical burr.
C. Normal clearance on the femoral neck is restored with removal of the bump.

There's a final step at the end of surgery: a dynamic test to make sure the bones are no longer impacting against each other. We take the foot out of the holder on the table and move the hip through flexion, extension, and rotation. We want to test how the hip is going to move in its native state, without traction. The camera is still inside the peripheral compartment so we can see this movement.

Today's surgery usually takes about an hour and a half. Once we've finished our work, we remove the instruments and the arthroscope. The two puncture sites are closed with one stitch for each. A sterile compressive dressing will be placed over the hip, and you'll be taken to the recovery room.

You will spend the same length of time in the recovery room as any other patient following more major surgery because your anesthesia has to wear off. If you need pain medication, it will be administered. You will go home the same day.

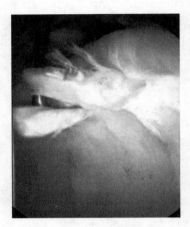

Photo 13-2. A torn, frayed labrum as seen through the scope during surgery.

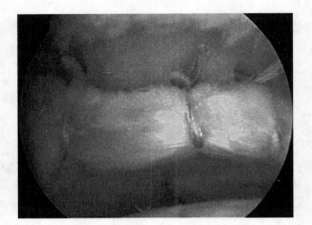

Photo 13-3. Sutures in place after labral repair.

Possible Complications

All surgical procedures have the risk of possible complications. You should understand them. Here are the most common possible complications you could face:

- Scar tissue
- Instability
- Potential femoral neck fracture
- Nerve problems
- Extra bone formation

Scar tissue

One of the biggest issues we face is the formation of scar tissue inside the joint. Bleeding sets off a healing cascade that creates scar tissue, and because we're shaving bone, this operation has a lot of exposed, bleeding bone inside the joint. We think this is part of the reason for the increased amount of scar tissue. Excess scarring can happen where we suture the labrum around the bony rim of the acetabulum or where we shave the bone formation off the femoral neck (cam). The capsule might adhere to those spots, which can mean that the hip becomes bound by scar tissue.

In many of these cases, the MRI looks normal—we can't see the scar tissue. But what we see when we get inside the joint can look like a sheet of scar tissue extending from the labrum to the femoral neck. We cut it, release it, and people get better because there's no bleeding bone this time around. We see a higher incidence of scar tissue formation in women than in men, possibly because of hormones.

Instability

We don't like to do arthroscopic surgery on patients who have dysplasia (a shallow socket) or loose ligaments around their hip joints because they can develop instability in the joint and dislocate the ball from the socket. But if we do the surgery, we take extra precautions. We will barely cut the capsule, maybe only a few millimeters, and after we repair the labrum, we'll use sutures to close the holes in the capsule. With most patients, we leave those openings intact to allow for easier movement. But with a "loosey-goosey" hip, we close all openings in the capsule to prevent instability.

Potential femoral neck fracture

The rule of thumb is that we can safely remove up to 25 percent of the bone from the femoral neck, but we take away much less than that. And we don't sculpt away bone any deeper than the native neck—the shape the femoral neck would have been if it hadn't had a defect. Although the chance of a fracture happening is extremely rare, it *has* happened, so we mention it for you to know. Those with osteoporosis and **osteopenia** would be the most at risk.

Nerve problems

You can experience nerve problems from traction or from the location of the incisions. As a result of traction, you can feel muscle weakness or numbness in your foot, calf, or other parts of your leg. Typically that resolves within seven days.

As a result of the incision, you may lose sensation in your leg from a nerve in the front of your thigh. The way that nerve branches out like a tree is different in every person. So when we cut your skin, some people get numbness at the front or side of the thigh—and some people don't. If you do get this numbness, it usually resolves.

Extra bone formation

During the surgery, we're shaving away pieces of bone from a cam or pincer bony formation. We are vacuuming out the bone as we operate, but we can't capture every single piece. Little particles can get imbedded in the muscle, and those could form extra bone if left untreated. So, for a month after surgery, we put patients on an anti-inflammatory like Advil or Aleve to prevent the bone from re-forming. Bone reformation happens through an inflammatory series of steps, so if you take anti-inflammatories, that stops the process.

Robots and CT Scans in Surgery

Navigation and computers may help us surgically shape a more perfect hip. We could take a CT scan or an MRI of a patient's hip and feed that data into the computer. There would be a sensor on the shaving tool to tell us where to shape. It would say, "shave, shave, shave," then it would tell us when we were finished so we would stop in exactly the right place. You would still need an experienced surgeon, but computer navigation is our first step in bringing robots into the OR. Their eyes are better than ours in seeing the precise amount of bone to remove.

Recovery from Arthroscopy

Even though you'll be icing and taking it fairly easy for the first two days, we do get you moving very quickly. The day after surgery, you'll ride a stationary bike and go for three short walks to your tolerance. You'll be keeping your bandage dry, typically for the first two days; then you can remove it, shower, and put Band-Aids over the two wounds.

The first night, your surgeon will give you a narcotic pain medication. We encourage patients to limit their narcotic use to the first night to prevent narcotic side effects such as constipation, lightheadedness, and upset stomach. We switch our patients to high-dose Advil, 600 milligrams, three times a day. This anti-inflammatory helps with pain and inflammation.

Your doctor will have you return to get the stitches out between seven and ten days after surgery. We don't use dissolvable stitches because the leg will become so swollen that it will put significant tension on the skin and those sutures could pop. We use a permanent nylon stitch that's stronger and will hold together. After the swelling calms down, it is still in place and needs to be removed. After that, you'll start physical therapy.

We don't want to create skin complications, so you should wait two weeks before you get into the pool. Then you can start deep-water running and other pool exercises for the first six weeks. If you're a swimmer, you can swim with a pull buoy between your legs (see page 301), but don't kick your legs until after the six-week mark. See chapter 16 on page 296 for a complete pool and land post-surgical program.

The magic number in orthopedics is six weeks—that's how long it takes for anything we have repaired to fully heal. That means your labrum heals about six weeks after surgery. We used to keep patients non–weight bearing for six weeks after removing cam bone off the femoral neck. We thought we were weakening the femoral neck, but we've learned that we can remove up to 25 percent of the femoral neck and still be fine. Since we're removing so much less than that, we no longer wait six weeks for bone to heal. But there *are* movement precautions in place to protect your new labrum. Don't do deep squats, deep lunges, straight leg raises, or clamshells until approved by your surgeon or therapist.

Gluteal Muscle/Flexor Muscle Imbalance

We've found a lot of data saying that people with FAI have gluteal muscle dysfunction—their gluteals aren't strong enough to be in balance with their opposing muscles, the hip flexors. They are like a drummer in a rock band who isn't keeping the right beat. It's hard for the rest of the band to play in sync without him. You probably had gluteal dysfunction before you ever met your surgeon, so now you have to get that drummer in sync with the rest of the band.

Your goal is to have your gluteal strength match your hip flexor strength. The gluteal muscles are at the back of your hip. They contract when you extend your hip, or reach your leg backward. The hip flexors contract when you flex your hip, or reach your leg forward. When the gluteals contract, the flexors must relax to allow movement; conversely, when the flexors fire, the gluteals must relax. (See a complete explanation of how muscles work in pairs on page 113.) Since you've had hip pain long enough to seek medical attention, you probably lost strength and function in your gluteal muscles. Now you must restore strength to restore the muscle balance.

After three months, you're likely to be feeling very good: you've gotten back your range of motion, your inflammation is down, and your labrum has healed. Everything has calmed down. Now your focus has to be on gluteal strength. It may take you six months to a year to regain gluteal strength and to get them working in a synchronous fashion with your other muscles. To a large degree, your recovery depends on how much time you put into your rehabilitation.

You might develop hip flexor tendinitis at the front of your hip during your recovery process. Don't think that because you have hip flexor pain as you exercise you're hurting your hip. It's normal at this stage of your rehabilitation. Don't hold back! We want you to continue exercising so you will eventually reach a point where you get enough gluteal muscle cells firing to strike a balance with the hip flexors. Then your hip will function more efficiently, and the pain in your hip flexors will diminish.

See chapter 16 for a pool and land rehab protocol that will guide you through the three phases of recovery after hip arthroscopy.

14

HIP IMPLANT SURGERY

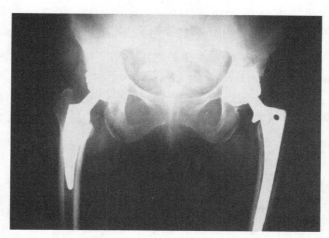

Figure 14-1. Implant X-ray. Notice how much smaller the new implant on the left is compared to the older one on the right.

This is the chapter we hoped you wouldn't have to read!

Some of you won't be having implant surgery because you earned increased strength and mobility using our pool and land exercises in chapters 9 and 12. Think back to the win-win concept we introduced in chapter 7, and congratulate yourself for achieving win number one. Your win goes to the root of who we are—an orthopedic surgeon and a water-rehab authority. Our goal was to have you read this book, turn your exercise routine around, and fall in love with the water. You learned that the Fountain of Youth is in the fountain. We're proud of all of you who earned that first win and the reprieve from surgery.

We're also proud of those of you who put forth a serious effort in a pool or land therapy program but who believe they have failed in reducing their hip pain. You have gotten stronger, and you are probably functioning at a higher level than before you started. But you can't change the fact that you no longer have a cushion between your ball and socket—your articular cartilage is too damaged, and now you can feel the bone grinding against bone. It possibly wakes you from a deep sleep in the night as you turn over in bed. You may have reached the point where putting on your shoes and socks is excruciating. Sex may have become virtually impossible not only due to pain but also because you have lost range of motion. (In fact, pain during sex is most likely the number-one reason patients finally decide to see a surgeon.) You are probably taking pain medication, and you have reached the point where you can neither face your daily physical activities nor sleep through the night.

Welcome to win number two! The fitness you gained in your attempt to prevent surgery will serve you well as you face the rigors of surgery. When it is time to resume your rehab exercises, you will be grateful that you've already learned them well prior to surgery. At a time when other things seem difficult following surgery, your familiar therapy exercises will come to you naturally. Since you honestly tried to go the conservative route, you will never have to second-guess yourself about whether you really needed the surgery or not.

If you are one of these patients, you'll find that knowing what takes place during implant surgery will make the operation less frightening to contemplate. Just as an athlete likes to walk the track, the field, or the court the night before a big competition, you can walk with me through the operating room (OR). By looking it all over, you should experience less fear and anxiety the day of your surgery.

More Hope for the Future

Technological advances continue to offer new hope and more options for people with hip problems, offering one more reason to try to postpone surgery. We all hope for a more elegant and holistic approach to solving hip problems, and every day brings us closer to it. It's possible that in five or ten years we might not be doing hip implant surgery. We can catch and treat arthritis sooner, we're looking at the creation of designer genes, and scientific solutions may provide more elegant options to address the structures that fail. I suspect we'll have a day soon when something totally unexpected will be created and we will say, "Wow, why didn't we think of *that* before?"

—Robert Klapper, MD

People commonly speak of total **hip replacement** surgery, but it is correctly called total **hip arthroplasty**. To be technically correct, we will call it hip implant surgery in this chapter. Although I perform surgery in Los Angeles, you can be assured that my hospital will be very similar to the hospital you'll be going to in Phoenix, Miami, New York, or anywhere else in the United States. Now let me be your surgeon for a chapter, and let me explain the many ways in which the old-fashioned hip replacement surgeries are now obsolete.

Types of Hip Implant Surgeries

You will probably be confused by many Internet websites and other sources of information regarding what the best approach is to the hip joint for your surgery. The joint can be reached through the back of the hip (posterior approach), the side of the hip (lateral approach), the front of the hip (anterior approach), or a combination of approaches. My personal preference, and the technique I'm most comfortable with, is called a posteriolateral approach—halfway between the back and the side. When I perform hip arthroscopy, I prefer the anterior approach.

My theory is that when surgeons stick with the technique they have mastered, they are less likely to end up with unfortunate outcomes or complications. So although you may hear about new surgical techniques, the most important thing is how comfortable your surgeon is with that technique. That's what I call the doctor's surgical preference. I don't want to dissuade you from having any particular approach; rather I wish to educate you on the options so you know what facts to consider for each.

The Posterior Approach

This has been the dominant surgical method for hip implant surgery for many years. The access to the hip is through an incision made close to the buttocks. This approach provides surgeons with a good view of the hip capsule, letting them easily place the implants in the correct positions and achieve equality of leg length.

Recently doctors have advanced this approach by reducing the size of the incisions and making it less invasive. We have also begun gently separating the muscles rather than cutting them. It's very simple: the less trauma we create in the muscles and surrounding tissues, the less pain the patient will feel and the more quickly they will heal.

The Lateral Approach

This was the first surgical approach used by Sir John Charnley, the British orthopedic surgeon who started the world of hip implant surgery. It remained his preferred approach throughout his career. In it, the patient is lying on his or her back, faceup on the table. The hip is entered by cutting the bone called the greater trochanter. This cut bone will later need to be repaired with wires. We are literally taking the hinges off the door to get into the house. You would never do that when you could just use the doorknob. But when the doorknob has been destroyed, you have to consider taking the hinges off to open the door.

The lateral approach is valuable when the destruction of the joint has twisted the bone severely or where scar tissue has made the other approaches to the joint more dangerous to the patient. It's been very rare in my career that I've used it, but I have it in my bag of tools of knowledge. Thus if the front door (anterior approach) is closed to me, and the back door (posterior approach) is closed to me, I can still get to the hip joint using the lateral approach. It is a great way to **revise** certain hips; but if it's not a revision, we generally try to do the posterior or anterior approach.

The Anterior Approach

During your research to find the right answer for your hip problem, you have probably read about the anterior approach for implant surgery. This is my preferred approach when I perform hip arthroscopy. Many doctors have begun performing implant surgery with this technique, which requires a special operating table and specialized tools. This table allows surgeons to move the leg through wide ranges of motion that typically are not possible when using a traditional operating table. However, the anterior approach also requires traction, which can lead to skin problems or a risk of numbness, tingling, or burning sensations along the thigh due to nerve problems. The reported advantage to this approach is that the surgeon encounters no muscles and can go directly from the skin into the hip capsule. But don't be confused: the capsule is still cut, and the joint still dislocated in order to perform the surgery.

Surgeons who perform this technique point to the fact that since the incision is in the front, you'll avoid the pain of sitting on the incision site. They also say leg length can be more accurate and that you'll have a quicker recovery. You should also know that most surgeons will require X-ray to guide them through the procedure. Ultimately what matters is your surgeon's preference and comfort with a given technique. If they do the anterior approach and have had predictable, successful results, then that's the approach you should take, in which case you will lie on your back on the table and your foot will be placed in a boot to allow for traction to be applied to your hip joint.

Now that you've read about the different approaches, be sure to ask your surgeon which approach he or she will be using and why. Our goal is to empower you with information. Don't be surprised if your surgeon is impressed with your research and knowledge.

Anesthesia Options

The selection of anesthesia is a major decision that you should discuss with your surgeon and anesthesiologist. There is **regional anesthesia** and **general anesthesia**. Regional anesthesia blocks the nerves to a specific area of the body. You remain conscious, so you will be given sedatives to relax you and put you into a light sleep. There are three kinds of regional anesthesia: a **nerve block**, an **epidural block**, or a **spinal block**. General anesthesia puts your whole body to sleep temporarily.

One of the greatest advances in hip surgery has been in the options you'll find for anesthesia. General anesthesia is still an option, but we are seeing it less and less. The side effects of those drugs, which delay the postoperative course—nausea, vomiting, and constipation—have made regional anesthesia the first choice for the modern hip surgery. Using it, you can hope for a quicker recovery after surgery.

Positioning the Patient

You'll be wheeled into the OR lying on your back. If you've been given a sedative, you most likely won't remember this. The anesthesiologist stands at the head of the table. He or she administers the anesthesia and monitors your vital signs throughout the surgery. The surgical equipment is at the opposite end of the room. Once the anesthetic has taken full effect, you will be positioned for surgery. Your surgeon may do things differently, but the hip surgery I do requires that the patient be placed on his or her side. We gently turn the patient so that the hip needing surgery is up. It's important for me to position my own patients rather than have the assistants do it for me because I want to make sure the patient isn't leaning one way or the other and is well supported with padding. We hold the patient in place with positioners on the OR table. These padded bumpers keep the patient in a fixed "home base" position so that while we're moving the leg during surgery, the pelvis and the rest of the body will remain locked in place.

If you are having a lateral approach surgery, you will be positioned faceup. For the anterior approach surgery, you will be transferred onto a specialized surgical table on your back and your foot will be placed in a boot to allow for the distraction of your hip joint.

Shaving, Sterilizing, and Dressing the Leg

If you have a fair amount of hair on your body, we shave the area where I'll be making the incision. The nurse uses an antiseptic solution to sterilize the entire leg. Even the toes are covered with antiseptic. Various drapes are placed so that your full body is covered. Next we wrap sterile dressings around the leg up to the site of the incision. This is an extra effort to minimize bacterial exposure of the wound. We want everything covered except the surgical site.

The Incision

The surgery that I am about to describe is my surgical preference. I've performed thousands of surgeries over the years and am comfortable with the anatomy so that I protect the nerve and make the leg lengths equal. I use a minimally invasive posterior approach.

I use a felt-tip marker to draw a line where I'm going to make the incision (Photo 14-1). The line for this patient is approximately three-and-a-half inches long and angled back into the buttocks, but if you have more fat below your skin, the incision will be longer. The cross marks on the skin help me close the wound correctly at the end of surgery. Without cross marks, it would be more difficult to line up the two ends of the wound—there could be a puckering or unevenness to the closure, as if you buttoned your shirt one button off. We will place clear plastic over the skin in this area to further sterilize the site before I make the incision.

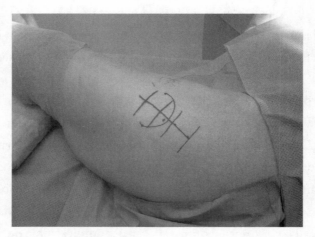

Photo 14-1. Dr. Klapper draws a line where he will make the incision. The reverse letter *C* is drawn around the greater trochanter, a surface landmark he uses to center the incision. You can see the greater trochanter in Drawing 2-1 on page 17.

We can make incisions so much shorter than we used to because we've learned to make a "mobile" opening that acts as a window into the hip joint. We can move the window up, down, forward, and back without having to cut the skin more than absolutely necessary. But if the tissues of a patient are too rigid and fixed so that the window isn't mobile, then we have to extend the incision or risk injury to the nearby nerve or artery. We must recognize we could do more harm by focusing strictly on the size of the incision.

If you have congenital causes for your hip problem or massive anatomical changes to your hip joint, this may be another reason that I would choose to make a larger, more accommodating incision. This would be better than possibly causing damage to the misshapen joint by forcing myself to work through an incision that is simply too small to get the job done correctly. Keep these factors in mind—a larger incision isn't necessarily an indictment of the surgeon's work.

Surgery: Minimally Invasive

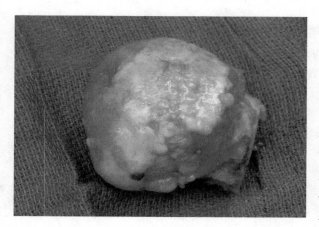

Photo 14-2. The defective, pitted ball (head of the femur) is removed.

When I compare today's surgery with the ones I learned at the beginning of my career, I'm amazed. Incisions used to be eight to ten inches long, whereas now they are three-and-a-half to four inches. The implants used to be six inches long; now they are three inches. The materials for the implants are harder and more durable and last longer. We have improved the incision; we have enhanced the materials; we have made the implant more customized. We have truly made this substantial surgery less invasive.

As we said before, you'll generally hear this operation called a total hip replacement, but I am not totally replacing your hip. I'm resurfacing the two sides of the joint, putting in new pieces to take the place of your faulty cartilage. My goal is to reproduce a frictionless surface on both sides of the joint.

When I've opened the hip joint, I carefully measure the dimensions of the ball so I know exactly what to restore. I remove the defective cartilage and the underlying bone, which means removing the entire head of the femur. (Photo 14-2 shows the pits and craters in the cartilage that ruined the smooth functioning of this hip.)

Next I prepare the shaft of the femur to accept the new implant. I create a tunnel in the soft marrow inside the bone that will match the shape of the implant, then put the implant snugly into place. We no longer use glue or cement to hold the implant in place. The implant has a rough surface called a porous coating, and the bone grows into that porous coating on the implant. We have learned that bone ingrowth into the implant requires fewer square inches of contact than we previously thought. Thus the implants can be smaller with even less coating.

On the socket side of the joint, I again take careful measurements before I start so we can recreate the same dimensions. I use what looks like a dome-shaped cheese grater to remove a potato-chip thickness of the cartilage from inside the socket. Then I prepare the bony bed to receive the new socket and choose the exact size metal hemisphere that will fit flawlessly into it. I gently tap the implant into place. Sometimes we use one screw to help hold it in place, but the screw isn't what's really holding it. It's the fact that the size is exactly right and it fits snugly in place. KlapperVision: It's like pushing one baseball hat into a second baseball hat.

The smaller, more customized implants have shortened the actual time of surgery. So have the smaller incisions. If we cut less, we have to repair less. At the start of my career, it took nearly two hours to perform this operation. Today it takes me a little more than thirty minutes.

Tranexamic acid (TXA)

A terrific advance is tranexamic acid, a new medicine we're using during the surgery. It's a liquid given either intravenously or placed directly onto the exposed muscles and tissues of the wound. This new medicine is actually an old medicine that was used in Canada. Since it's been around a long time and is fully acknowledged as a safe drug, I know I won't end up apologizing for side effects we didn't anticipate. In the past few years, it has become the standard of practice in the operating room at leading hospitals that perform hip implant surgeries.

In essence, it allows surgical bleeding, even a small amount of bleeding, to clot and stay clotted so that bleeding doesn't continue into the wound later. Don't be confused by the two kinds of blood clots. We want to stop bleeding at the surgical site, so we're glad TXA keeps those clots in place. But at the same time, we're also worried about blood clots forming in a vein in either of your legs. We give people blood thinners to prevent those clots. You'll read on pages 277 to 278 about the importance of preventing the dangerous kind of clot that can flow up to the lung, making it impossible for you to breathe. But now we're referring to a local clot that is created due to surgery. TXA is a different medicine for that local wound. It's not going to create blood clots in your veins. By using TXA during surgery, we have less bleeding in the surgical wound, which means less pressure, less swelling, and therefore less pain. Even more importantly, there will be less bleeding the next day and the day after that. Because of this, we no longer have drains installed in the wound to remove excess bleeding.

> ### Another Benefit of TXA
>
> TXA stops bleeding, so there's less swelling, and therefore less pain. This gives patients a more comfortable post-operative experience because of less tension on the wound from the swelling. I can't prove it yet, but I believe that since there is less oozing from the wound due to TXA, we will see a decrease to the already-low incidence of infection.
>
> —Robert Klapper, MD

Custom-Making Your Implant

Not long ago, we had only small, medium, and large implants, and the surgeon had to chip away the patient's bone to fit the implant. Now we fit the patient's bone exactly. We use tools to measure inside the joint at the time of surgery. Thus we can create the perfect-sized implant for a basketball player who is seven feet tall as well as a jockey who is five feet tall—and it's all done during the surgery. Because the pieces of the implant come in various lengths, widths, and sizes, we're able to fit them together in various combinations, creating a large number of options.

In the OR, I have to sense what to do artistically that will give each patient the most **aesthetic** movement. I look at the quality of the bone and make the decision about the amount of porous coating that needs to be on the implant. This coating is a roughened surface that fools the body into thinking it is bone marrow, and the bone marrow cells grow right into this implant and hold it in place. The implant for some patients will be covered from top to bottom with porous coating; for others, I might choose an implant that isn't fully covered. We don't want more bony ingrowth than we need. If too much bone grows in, it will change the forces around the hip, which can create a limp or lead to other problems with the bone some years later. This is where the intuitive artist has to realize what's needed.

KlapperVision: Hard or Soft Bone

Let's imagine that I'm looking at a block of Styrofoam from a distance. It looks like a white cube on a table. If a white cube of marble of the same size is placed on the table next to it, I have no idea of the differences between the two cubes. That's the way it feels when I'm looking at bone on an X-ray, like looking from a distance. But as I get closer, I realize that I could stick my finger through the Styrofoam, but not the marble. That's what I experience during surgery, when I get a firsthand look at the quality of the bone. For me to choose the correct pieces for the patient's implant, I have to assess two areas of the bone. What is the crackability and stiffness of the outside of the bone, the **cortex**? What is the mushiness or thickness of the marrow inside the bone? As soon as I use the saw to take off the cartilage, I know if it is hard or soft bone. I can tell by how the blade feels in the bone. It would be as if you cut either a frozen or a fresh loaf of bread. You would know right away.

When I encounter the equivalent of Styrofoam bone, I'm going to use a fatter, thicker, more-coated implant. If I encounter the marble, I'll use a thinner, smaller, less-coated implant. By and large, the harder bone is the healthier bone. Hard bone will latch completely onto the implant, so I don't need a lot of porous coating.

–Robert Klapper, MD

Next I choose the correct ball size to go onto the head of the femur. This is the main place to adjust leg lengths. Choose the wrong one, and there could be a leg-length discrepancy after surgery. I focus on returning the leg lengths exactly to where they started. However, there is a complication you should know about: I may have to make a judgment call during your surgery.

Picture the cartilage of your hip joint. Let's say that before you had arthritis, the cartilage was one-half-inch thick on the ball side of the joint and one-half-inch thick on the socket side of the joint. That made a combined thickness of one inch of cartilage. As arthritis caused the deterioration of your cartilage, the thickness may have decreased by, let's say, half, so you now have only one-half-inch thickness of total cartilage. Now picture your ligaments, the static stabilizers that cross the joint. They were pulled tight, stabilizing your hip. They were used to the one-half inch plus one-half inch that equaled one inch. But as your cartilage wore away, your ligaments didn't shrink to maintain their tautness since they now only span one-fourth inch plus one-fourth inch, equaling one-half inch. So the stabilizers can't do their job, and the joint can feel unstable. During surgery, if I see that your ligaments no longer stabilize your hip joint, I will have to lengthen your leg to recreate that tautness so that your hip won't be unstable and dislocate. Your surgeon, too, may have to decide to give you a leg-length discrepancy to protect you from dislocations. Although this happens rarely, it is a factor that surgeons must consider in every single surgery.

The implant consists of the following pieces:

The ball. There are different ball sizes since this is the main place where I adjust the leg length. Ball size #1 versus ball size #4 can provide an extra inch in the overall length of the leg. The diameter, or width of the ball, can be the size of a Ping-Pong ball, a smooth golf ball, or a tennis ball. Having various sizes and diameters helps me recreate the correct anatomy. The ball can be metal or ceramic.

The femoral component. This implant is the **titanium metal alloy** piece that fits into the shaft of your femur. It comes in various widths and lengths, so a correct size can be chosen to create the right implant to fit your bone. The ball fits onto the end of the implant, in effect becoming the new head of your femur. This connection is the Morse Taper as explained in the box on p. 262.

The socket. We also have different sizes and choices for the socket side of the joint. A metal shell with porous coating locks into the surgically-prepared bone of the acetabulum. Into that shell is placed a plastic or ceramic liner. Again, picture pushing one baseball hat into a second baseball hat.

By judging the quality of the bone correctly and carefully choosing each of the pieces of the implant, we're able to build for each individual the most durable, efficient new hip joint possible and restore his or her anatomy perfectly.

Bearing Surfaces

When we speak of bearing surfaces, we're speaking of the materials we implant on the ball-and-socket side of the joint. When you walk, those two surfaces meet. Those are your weight-bearing, or bearing, surfaces. Will your new hip be made of metal against plastic? Is it ceramic against plastic? Is there no plastic, but metal-on-metal?

I have chosen through my career to use primarily metal against plastic. I have avoided using ceramic as a bearing surface except in rare cases of a patient who has a metal allergy. Nickel is the primary metal that is problematic. If you can't wear jewelry because of a metal allergy, your doctor may send you to an allergist who can get powdered nickel and titanium for a skin test.

The recent recall of metal against metal implants is because of the high failure rate of this operation. Some instinct kept me away from using that in hip implant surgeries. I have also avoided using ceramic as a bearing surface. I have done so because I have stuck with technology that has been extremely successful and predictable. I didn't know that some patients with ceramic or metal-on-metal implants would have hips that squeak. Nor did I know that in rare cases of ceramic implants cracking, the revision surgery is quite difficult because there are many pieces of ceramic in the surrounding soft tissues. These complications are reasons I've been happy I did not stray to these other bearing surfaces.

I've always felt strongly that medicine is not controversial at all if you pretend the patient you're about to operate on is your own mother. That has been my guiding principle through my career. Your surgeon may have different thoughts; I can only speak to mine. In my hands, the use of metal against plastic has had the most predictable and best outcomes.

Femoral Head Resurfacing (The Birmingham Hip)

Many surgeons have had the idea that anchoring an implant into the thigh bone was more surgery than necessary. They pictured capping the ball with a new metal surface instead of cutting through the bone and removing the head of the femur. This procedure has been performed in Europe for several decades and was recently FDA-approved in the United States. It is called femoral head resurfacing, and I performed many of these surface replacements in the recent past because I believed it to be a worthwhile procedure for a young, active male. The problem with doing it for females is that they are more likely to have osteoporosis, which makes the incidence of fractures in these cases unacceptable. I would do the surgery only on males between twenty and sixty. Men older than that can also develop osteoporosis and be at risk of bone fracture.

The downside is that this surgery requires more trauma to the soft tissues than doing a traditional hip implant. When we remove the femoral head and neck in traditional hip implant surgery, we are then able to see more of the anatomy that's deeper, allowing us better visibility because we have removed that bone. Ironically, when we do a surface replacement surgery, which removes less bone, we need to open a bigger wound to do the surgical work. So the surgery that is less invasive on the bone is actually more invasive on the soft tissue.

Patients were willing to live with that extra soft-tissue trauma if it meant they retained more of their own bones. But then we began to learn that the long-term complications of metal-on-metal may make this bearing surface unacceptable. The metal can begin to wear, shedding small particles of metal debris that can be absorbed into nearby tissues or enter the bloodstream. We have seen this create inflammatory reactions that can cause pain in the groin and destruction of the soft tissue and bone around the hip. Women are far more likely than men to be affected in this way.

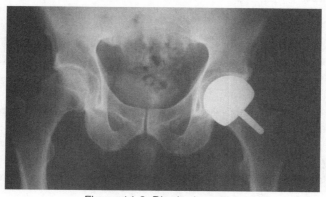

Figure 14-2. Birmingham hip.

It's important for surgeons to have this option available for some of their patients. For instance, I did this operation on a twenty-one-year-old male. At age eight, he was involved in a terrible accident, and his femur grew looking more like a pretzel than a pipe. The surface replacement was the perfect operation in his case because I couldn't create an implant to fit down the shaft of his misshapen femur. Now he's a happy young man because he can finally walk without pain or a limp. That's why I believe it's good for surgeons to have this in their tool bag—and in the future, I expect the metal-on-metal issues to be resolved, and I will once again be doing it routinely.

Dual Mobility Implants

This is a fantastic item to have in the tool bag—it can work beautifully for patients who need revisions or those with chronic dislocations. This implant has three major pieces instead of two. Instead of a ball in a socket, this implant adds another socket floating just inside the rigid socket we described above. Normally, we put metal inside the socket and the ball is made of plastic. With the dual mobility implant, the rigid socket is still metal, but the large floating socket is plastic. The large size of this floating socket has brought down the risk of dislocation to almost zero. The inner ball is made of either metal or ceramic.

With great stability, little threat of dislocation, and dramatically increased range of motion, why don't we want to use this with all our hip implant surgeries? Because it doesn't duplicate the normal feel and biomechanics of our hip joints. As human beings, we have only two moving parts in our hips, not three. There's probably a good reason for that. Also, the implant might not last as long as our tried-and-true ones, but we won't know that for many more years. Thus I would use this implant for someone who has had problems with dislocations, but I would not use it as a first choice for a hip unless it was being revised.

Closing the Incision

When the surgical work is complete, I immediately begin closing the wound using sutures to bring the various deep tissues together. Once we're near the skin, I close the majority of patients with absorbable stitches that are placed just below the surface of the skin. These stitches do not need to be removed. The body will resorb them on its own. I use a plastic surgical closure, meaning that as I advance the needle from side to side of the open skin, I do it as meticulously as the work performed by plastic surgeons. The cross marks (shown in Photo 14-1 on page 256) guide me so I can precisely restore the edges of the incision. Next I place a liquid adhesive on top to make the skin sticky, and on top of that I place Steri-Strips, a series of small paper Band-Aids.

When a patient has a great amount of fat at the incision site, that fat can die, leading to a liquid formation below the skin called fat **necrosis**. That liquid can prevent the healing from occurring properly. If the skin is slow to heal, this liquified fat will seep out of the wound and can lead to an infection by creating a pathway for germs to enter the wound. So where there's extra fat, I use retention sutures that reach deeper and bring more of the fatty skin edges together. I also add staples to create a firmer seal. This combats slow healing, but these sutures and staples or clips need to be removed in the office.

Obesity is the Number-One Cause of Wound-Site Infection

Obesity, a national epidemic, has been shown in recent papers to be the number-one cause of wound-site infection following hip surgery. It's not HIV; it's not diabetes. It's obesity. You should make this your biggest motivating reason to lose excess weight before having hip surgery.

—Robert Klapper, MD

When Surgery Is Over

The patient is gently returned to a position lying on his or her back. Inflatable foot pumps are placed around both the patient's feet and ankles, like socks with air in them. You'll learn more about the benefits of foot pumps and how they work in chapter 15.

Even though I do everything in my power to help my patients prevent or delay surgery for as long as possible, when it's time for the hip implant, I encourage them to look forward to an improved quality of life. Hip surgery is one of the reasons I'm so passionate about orthopedics because I'm taking one of the most debilitating, life-interrupting problems that can happen to people and giving them their lives back.

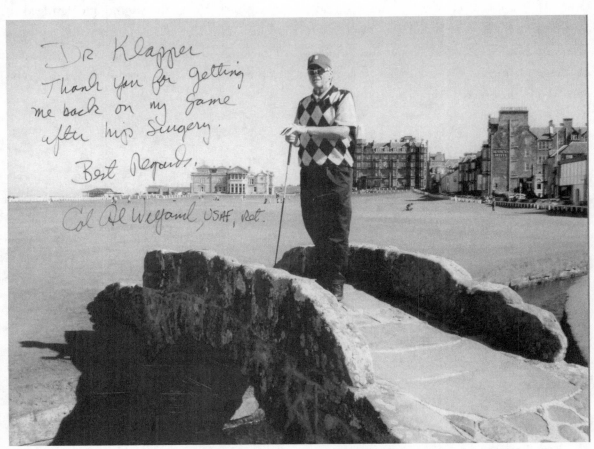

Dr Klapper
Thank you for getting
me back on my game
after hip surgery.

Best Regards,

Col Al Wiegand, USAF, Ret.

Photo 14-7. Retired Air Force colonel, Al Wiegand, golfing at St. Andrews, Scotland.

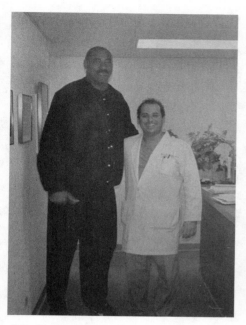

Wilt Chamberlain with Dr. Klapper, 1994.

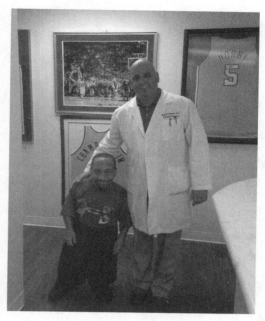

Tony Cox, actor, with Dr. Klapper, 2015.

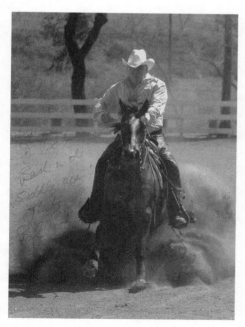

William Shatner, actor.

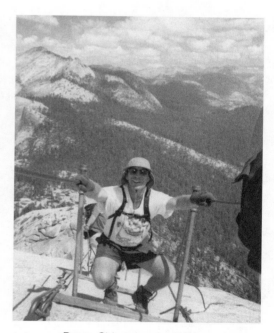

Bruce Shien, teacher hiking
Half Dome, Yosemite.

15

IN AND OUT OF THE HOSPITAL

If you've never had an operation or never spent time in a hospital, you'll have dozens of questions, concerns, and, yes, fears as you prepare for hip implant surgery. In this chapter we'll try to allay your fears and concerns by giving you so much information that you'll feel like a veteran on arrival at the hospital.

One of the first things you can do is talk directly to another of your surgeon's patients who has successfully gone through the whole process. I make that easy in my office by having a list of patients who have given me permission to give out their phone numbers and who are good at talking about what happened to them. I've got a range of ages and personality types on the list, so if I have a patient who is an active woman in her forties who wants to return to skiing, I look at my list and match her up with someone with similar concerns and goals. I match women with women and men with men, and I do my best to match their diagnoses exactly. If you have a fracture, arthritis, a congenital problem, or an additional back problem, you should speak to someone else with the same condition who has gone through the same surgery.

A patient may have questions she isn't comfortable discussing with me, such as "When can I get up by myself to go to the bathroom again?" or "When can I have sex again?" It's also important for patients to ask such questions as, "Am I going to be able to reach my doctor by phone after surgery?", "Is his or her bedside manner genuine?", and "What was your relationship like with the doctor in terms of care before, during, and after the surgery?" Talking these things over with an "experienced" patient who used the same surgeon as you can provide much more valuable information and reassurance than the generalities you will find on the Internet.

Prior to Surgery

Between the time your surgery is scheduled and the date of the surgery itself, there are several things you can do to help ensure the best possible outcome.

You Might Donate Blood

We used to have patients donate two pints of blood in the weeks leading up to their surgery, and we often used at least one of those pints during the surgery to replace lost blood. But with today's advancements in the surgery, you'll lose very little blood, so your surgeon may not have you donate any blood at all. I still have patients donate one pint of blood because there's no question that the safest blood to receive if you lose blood during surgery is your own. From my point of view, the blood is there just in case of an emergency. I may ultimately phase this out completely, but this is my current practice.

If your surgeon says you will be donating blood, find out which blood bank works with your hospital and contact it. A transfusion specialist will see you and go over the details. Generally the blood can be stored for about six weeks before surgery.

Visit an Internist or Your Family Doctor

Although internists, family practice doctors, and general practitioner doctors are slightly different, all three of them look at your overall medical condition. About two weeks before your scheduled operation, you'll have a general physical exam to make sure that you're a safe candidate for surgery. The doctor will test your heart and lungs and take blood tests and a chest X-ray. All of these pre-op tests make sure you're fit for the surgery.

Before you visit the doctor, prepare a typed or clearly printed list of all your medications, including the dose and the frequency. Add all the vitamins and supplements you take as well. Your doctor will decide which medications and supplements might need to be stopped prior to surgery and which to continue. We have seen gingko biloba increase bleeding and vitamin K increase the risk of blood clots. You may consider the things you take to be natural, but they can possibly affect your surgery, so disclose all of them. You will also want to discuss with your doctor any allergies you have to medications or food.

If you drink alcohol regularly, inform your doctor how many drinks you have a day or if you recently quit drinking. Do the same regarding smoking: tell your doctor the number of cigarettes you smoke a day, or if you recently quit smoking. Inform your doctor if you use recreational drugs—give the names of the drugs, how often you use them, or if you have recently quit such use.

If you don't have your own medical doctor, or if your doctor doesn't practice at your surgeon's hospital, your surgeon should recommend one for you.

Take a Pre-Op Education Class

Not all hospitals have a pre-op education class. If yours doesn't, you'll actually get a mini-version of such a class right here in this chapter, a comprehensive preview of what's to come. If your hospital does have a pre-op class, it is extremely helpful to attend it. You will most likely meet a surgical nurse, a physical therapist, and an anesthesiologist who will talk you through your entire stay in the hospital. You'll learn about anesthesia, painkillers, and the use of assistive walking devices. If you will have hip precautions (see page 284), they will be discussed to prepare you for the coming restrictions in your movements.

Research shows that patients who attend a presurgical education class are discharged from the hospital sooner than those who do not attend. They know what to expect, so they handle it better—and that includes handling pain. The class also helps eliminate the shock some patients experience when they're asked to get out of bed so quickly after surgery. If they're unprepared for such a request, some of them will say, "What do you mean I have to get up the very same day?" Research shows patients have to get upright almost immediately for optimal recovery.

Prepare Your Home for Your Return

Especially if you live alone, you must have your things prepared in advance. Think about what things you have to bend over for in your daily life. Move them to a higher position. Consider having meals already prepared and in your freezer and groceries in your cupboards. Move comfortable clothes to the front of your closet.

Think of other ways you can make your home more convenient to live in upon your return. Have your favorite pillows handy. You'll be more comfortable with a pillow between your legs both in bed and at other times during your recovery, and you will promote good scarring. If your chairs at home are low, pile one cushion onto another to give you height. Following hip precautions, including sitting in a higher chair, is still relevant for your first six weeks.

Understand Your Insurance Benefits

During your stay in the hospital, you'll want to devote your time and effort to healing. This means you should do all the research about your insurance well before your operation.

Many of today's health plans use various "networks," groups of health-care providers that contract with your hospital. Your surgeon and the hospital you choose may both be part of your network, but many of the services they'll use are not. The anesthesiologist is a medical doctor who administers and supervises the anesthesia, the drugs that will sedate you or make you unconscious. The anesthesiologist who usually works in the operating room with your surgeon might not be part of your network. The lab that does your urine and blood work might not be either. If you go blindly into surgery without researching, you'll receive bills from companies you've never heard of after the surgery. Many of them won't be part of your network and that will trigger a different, and probably higher, deductible on your insurance.

You should take the time to find out exactly what services you'll need for the surgery and what companies you can select that are part of your network. This can save you hundreds of dollars. You may, however, decide to keep your doctor's "team" together. For instance, if the anesthesiologist who usually works with your surgeon in the operating room isn't in your network, you may decide that their close working relationship is worth the extra money.

In particular, you should know what your post-hospital benefits are. Does your insurance pay for home care or another extended care facility? Your doctor wants you well taken care of, and he or she might say, "Since you don't have anyone at home to help, we'll send you to this place." But your insurance may not pay for the place your doctor has in mind.

Find out what equipment your insurance will pay for. The physical therapists will teach you how to use a walker or cane safely. You'll continue to need an assistive walking device when you first leave the hospital. Many insurance companies will pay for only one walking device, so don't buy anything prior to surgery. Let the physical therapist decide with you on the best type of equipment specifically for you. In your room, you'll use a high toilet seat for comfort and safety, and you may want to have one for home use also. The occupational therapist will teach you to use a reaching device so you won't have to bend over to pick things up from the floor. The therapists will teach you tricks using this "reacher" so you can safely put on your shoes and socks or pick up things you drop. The hospital staff will do their best to verify what will be paid for by your insurance, but you should know too. If they send you home with equipment that won't be paid for by your insurance, you will be paying for it.

Other Preparations

Every hospital is different. Some have private rooms, others have two or more patients per room. Some have satellite TV, some don't. Do your research well ahead of surgery if those details concern you. You'll want to avoid a major surprise during the crucial days of recovery in the hospital.

Remember that list of medications that you prepared for the internist? Bring a copy of it with you to the hospital. Your medications will be provided by the hospital during your stay, and the staff will make sure you continue to take them appropriately. List all your allergies to medicine and food.

Report any health changes since your presurgical physical exam to your surgeon. Inform your surgeon of any cuts, scrapes, or sores on your affected leg. Tell your surgeon if you have any signs of infection, such as chills, fever, coughing, or a runny nose within a week of your scheduled surgery.

You will be instructed to bathe with Chlorhexedine soap the night before surgery and the morning of surgery. Research studies show this helps prevent postoperative infections. Your doctor's office will supply it or tell you where you can obtain a bottle.

You must stop eating and drinking by midnight the night before surgery. Keeping your stomach empty reduces nausea and vomiting in case the drugs don't agree with you. However, follow the instructions from your doctor about taking any of your daily medications with sips of water early on the morning of your surgery. Blood pressure pills are a good example of meds you will take.

Day of Surgery: Check-In

Most patients are asked to check-in to the hospital the day of surgery, two hours before the scheduled time of the operation. Operating rooms generally open around 7:30 a.m., so your arrival time might be quite early. You should find out about parking in advance. You don't want to be late because you couldn't find a parking place.

Wear casual, loose-fitting clothing that won't press against your incision site on your return home. Wear a comfortable pair of shoes that you can slip into easily without bending to put them on.

You'll start at the admissions office. The admissions desk will have a list of all the people who are having surgery that day, so they'll be expecting you. Study the following checklist. Then when you talk to that other patient who has had surgery similar to yours, ask if there was anything unique about your particular hospital. Was there anything he or she forgot to bring from home that would have made the hospital stay more pleasant?

Checklist: What to Take to the Hospital

- A list of the medications you're currently taking and the amount you take daily of each. Don't bring the actual medications with you. The hospital will supply them for you.
- Pajamas, a robe, slippers, glasses, hearing aid, dentures, and personal toiletries such as your toothbrush, hairbrush, shampoo, and deodorant.
- Insurance information.
- Emergency phone numbers.
- Your cane, crutches, or walker if you use them. Label them with your name. If they're misplaced while you're in surgery, they can easily be returned to you.
- A copy of your advance directives. These are written statements such as a living will or health-care power of attorney. They communicate your wishes for your health care if you are unable to communicate those wishes for yourself. Advance directives forms are usually available through your hospital.
- *Don't* bring anything of value into the hospital the day of surgery. You don't want to lose something you cherish. If you do bring valuable items, they will be locked up during your surgery and returned to you when you are transferred to your room.
- Bring only a few dollars in cash. Don't bring credit cards with you, but you can list your credit card number in a safe place along with the expiration date and three-digit security code.
- If you plan on bringing in your cell phone or laptop, you will find that most hospitals offer guest Internet services.
- Leave all jewelry at home.

Day of Surgery: Admission

A hospital employee or volunteer will take you to your next stop, a room in which you prepare for surgery. A nurse will admit you and review any requests your surgeon may have made.

At this point you will change into your hospital gown. It will button or tie in the back. Your clothes will be placed in a bag. If someone is with you, this is when you'll give him or her all your belongings, including your cell phone, wristwatch, rings, and other jewelry that you forgot to leave at home. If you're alone, your bag will be locked in a special closet until you've arrived in your room after surgery. Later that day these belongings will be brought to you.

Now that you're in your hospital gown, you'll wait until the surgical staff is ready for you. One of the reasons you're asked to be at the hospital two hours prior to your surgery is that if someone else's surgery is cancelled at the last minute, you could be whisked off into the operating room (OR) early. On the other hand, an operation might take longer than was expected, and you could go into surgery late. The timing of your surgery depends on what happens to the patients before you in your designated operating room. More than one surgeon may be sharing the room that day, so the timing doesn't always depend on your doctor alone. When it's time, you'll be taken to the pre-op holding area, and your family will be shown to the waiting room.

Day of Surgery: The Pre-Op Holding Room

A hospital employee will pick you up approximately forty-five minutes before your surgery is expected to begin. You'll be taken by wheelchair to pre-op, a holding room near the operating room. There the surgical staff will settle you onto a gurney (a stretcher on wheels) and make final preparations for surgery. The nurses in the pre-op room will introduce themselves. They'll always tell you what they're going to do before they do it.

If you wear glasses, contact lenses, a hearing aid, or dentures, you'll keep all of these in place until the last minute. In the past, nurses took everything from you that was removable, but now physicians and nurses want the patients to be as comfortable as possible—talking, hearing, and seeing until just before the surgery. Glasses and hearing aids are labeled with the patient's name and returned right after the surgery.

If your contact lenses are disposable, throw them away in pre-op. Bring your glasses because you may not feel well enough to put contacts in your eyes the first few days.

Your anesthesiologist will talk to you about your past surgical history and medical history. If you've had trouble with nausea or vomiting after anesthesia, this is the time to speak up because you can receive anti-nausea medication to reduce your chance of reoccurrence. If this is your first surgery, but you easily get carsick or seasick, you should also share this with your anesthesiologist. It will be helpful to discuss whether you have difficulty with controlling chronic pain conditions or if you've been taking pain medications at home. The anesthesiologist will discuss the different types of anesthesia available, namely general and regional anesthesia. In both situations you are completely asleep during the surgery. General anesthesia is a very deep state of anesthesia in which assistance with breathing is required, whereas regional anesthesia numbs a region of your body while a light sedative medication keeps you asleep. For hip surgery, if you have regional anesthesia, you will be numb from the waist down for a few hours. Many practitioners favor regional rather than general anesthesia since it has fewer side effects and faster recovery; however, your type of anesthesia should be determined based on a comprehensive evaluation of your past medical history, personal preference, and a thorough discussion with your anesthesiologist and surgeon.

The anesthesiologist will place a needle in your arm to begin the intravenous fluids. You'll hear this referred to as an IV. The fluids are composed of a potassium and saltwater solution called saline. The purpose of the IV is to give you the fluids your body would normally have or need. If your doctor ordered it, the anesthesiologist will give you a dose of antibiotics **prophylactically**. Your IV fluids will be stopped by the morning after surgery, but the IV access is usually kept in your arm in case you need more medications, fluids, or blood.

Just prior to surgery, I always come visit my patients. I follow several precautions. I know patients have only one gall bladder, but they have two hips, knees, and shoulders. I always ask them, "Which side are we doing today?" And I intentionally ask them how their other side is doing. Patients can be nervous and can grunt or nod their answers, so it's important for us to discuss their other side. I want them to say, "We're not doing my left hip; we're doing my right." I have another double-check in place. Even in this world of electronic medicine, where everything is in the computer, I still have my office print out the history and physical from the first day I saw the patient in my office. Errors can occur in medicine when everyone talks only about what they assume is the correct side. So I hand-carry my patients' charts to see that on a different date in the past, they came to me for right hip pain, not left hip pain. I do everything possible before every surgery to ensure that no mistakes are made.

I don't think there is any more powerful drug than laughter before surgery. For twenty-six years, I have told every one of my patients before surgery, "Don't forget, my father was a carpenter, and he taught me to measure twice, cut once." It always brings a smile or a chuckle from the patient and family members. I believe we'll learn in the future that the power of smiling and laughing prior to a stressful procedure somehow modulates the immune system in a positive way.

Someone from the surgical staff will pick you up from pre-op. They'll wheel you on your gurney into the operating room. If you're having general anesthesia, you won't remember much of this part because the anesthesiologist will have already started giving you medicine to calm you and start to put you to sleep.

Preventing Blood Clots

There are inherent risks of undergoing surgery, and you need to discuss them with your doctor. There's the risk that you could have a negative reaction to the anesthesia. There's the risk of damage to the nerves or the blood vessels since we're working so close to them. There's the risk that your leg lengths could differ from each other after the surgery. There's the risk of infection. But of all the possible complications that can happen from surgery, the most important is a blood clot, because it can kill you.

When we talk about a dangerous type of blood clot, we're talking about a clot developing in a vein in either of your legs. It sits there and then all of a sudden—right after surgery, the next day, a week later, a month later, or three months later—it lets loose and throws itself into the bloodstream and flows up to the lung. The blood clot lodges there and blocks off a part of the breathing area of that lung. If it's a big clot, you can try to breathe all you want, but there won't be an exchange of oxygen and you could die.

A blood clot in a vein is called a deep vein thrombosis (DVT), while a clot that travels from one place to another is called an embolism. A clot that sticks in the lung is called a pulmonary embolism. No matter what they're called, we want to avoid all of them, so we take many precautions. We try to thin the blood immediately after surgery with an injected blood thinner. Your surgeon will decide if you need to continue such medication in pill form when you go home. I currently enjoy using the **protocol** from the Hospital for Special Surgery in New York. I have patients take 325 milligrams of adult aspirin twice a day with food for a month or two after surgery. Recognize that this is my vote, but this decision is left to your surgeon.

During surgery, we use various medications to keep a patient's blood pressure low, and we try to finish the surgery quickly. After surgery, we try to get the patient upright as soon as possible. We use foot pumps, which are placed on both your feet in the operating room and are attached to an air pump machine. The pressure from the air pumps push against the balls of your feet making you involuntarily lift your toes. This mimics the act of walking and helps pump your blood back to your heart. The foot pumps keep your blood circulating so it doesn't collect in your veins and stagnate. At the same time, they create a chemical response to thin your blood. Studies show that foot pumps prevent a large number of clots during the first seventy-two hours after surgery. Ask your doctor what his or her routine is or what the hospital staff does.

The Body's Own Internal Pharmacy

More and more studies are showing the incredible value of using foot pumps. We're learning that these mechanical devices elicit a chemical response by the body that becomes a natural, self-made blood thinner. Just as beta-endorphin is your own body's pain medication, there are beneficial chemicals that your body makes to thin the blood, and they are created in reaction to the foot pumps.

I'm looking forward to the day when we will no longer use **pharmacology** for thinning of the blood, but instead use the body's own internal pharmacy. I hope it will be in the near future when I will embrace a protocol that has no oral or injectable medication.

—Robert Klapper, MD

After hip surgery, you'll have swelling in your ankle, your knee, and maybe your whole leg because we've blocked the normal flow of fluids upstream. The swelling could last for days, weeks, or even months. During that time, you'll probably want to buy some support stockings to help manage the swelling.

Pillows

By the time most people have hip surgery, they're usually already comfortable with a pillow between their legs as they sleep, so the introduction of such a pillow shouldn't be an intrusion. The pillow keeps your legs apart in a stable position for comfort and for non-disruption of the healing tissues and incision.

You may decide that you want the comfort of a pillow from home. If you do bring your own pillow, put a colored pillowcase on it, something that will distinguish it from the hospital's pillows. Without something to make it look different, your pillow could easily get mixed up with those at the hospital.

Pain Management

Pain can be scary, but today there are many options to help control surgical pain. Hospital staff members use a pain scale from zero to ten, with ten being the worst pain ever. The scale can be divided roughly into mild pain (one to four), moderate pain (five to seven), and severe pain (eight to ten). You will be asked to assess your pain level with a number; then the staff will medicate you based on that number. The physician prescribes different pain medications or doses for mild, moderate, and severe pain. It may be difficult to quantify your pain on a scale, but it's the most effective way to communicate with your doctors and nurses so they can treat your pain with precision.

The nurses will try to use oral medications to control the pain as much as possible so that you are able to be awake and not too drowsy. It is best to keep taking the pain medication every three to four hours so that the pain is controlled well. It is also a good idea to plan ahead with your nurse to take a pain pill forty-five minutes before your physical therapy sessions.

If the pain is not controlled well with oral medications, there are other options available such as IV medication, **patient-controlled analgesia** (**PCA**), nerve blocks, and epidurals. Nerve blocks and epidurals can offer pain relief directly to the pain fibers without increasing side effects often experienced with oral or IV pain medication. All of these options should be discussed with the surgeon.

Ice is used as a means to decrease pain and swelling. It can be ordered as ice packs applied to the surgical area or an ice machine that supplies continuous ice therapy. Both methods are effective. You can continue using ice at home to help alleviate pain.

Day of Surgery: In Your Room

From the operating room, you'll be taken to the recovery room. The nurses there and your anesthesiologist will decide when it's time for you to be moved to your hospital room for the rest of your stay. Your IV will still be in place. You'll probably be given a few more doses of antibiotics through it.

General anesthesia can give you a dry mouth and a feeling of being dehydrated. Patients who have regional anesthesia seem to wake up faster and are not usually nauseated. Some patients have no side effects at all and are hungry right after surgery. They can actually start eating in the recovery room. Most patients, however, will start with liquids first, then advance fairly quickly. Their first meal might be dinner the same evening of surgery.

Your bed will have a frame around it and a trapeze overhead. The trapeze is a bar you can grasp with your hands so you can use your arms to help adjust the position of your body. As you progress, you'll use it to get in and out of bed.

Right after surgery, the nurses will ask you to do some ankle pumps: they'll say, "Push your toes away, then pull them back toward your head." They want to make sure you have control of your muscles and that all of the nerves are functioning. Also, ankle pumps help blood flow in the legs.

You'll need to take some deep breaths to keep your lungs working well. The number-one reason why some people have a fever right after surgery is a collapse of the small airways in the lungs. That collapse can cause a fever that could lead to pneumonia if not managed correctly. You need a good expansion of your lungs, and just being told to breathe deeply isn't enough. An **incentive spirometer** is a device created to motivate patients to breathe deeply. Essentially it's a plastic toy. You'll use your own breath to move three balls to the top of the device and hold them there for a few seconds. You get visual feedback about how deeply you can breathe and hold that deep breath. You'll do that several times an hour whenever you're awake. It's a wonderful way to keep your lungs clear following the anesthesia required for surgery. If using a spirometer isn't a normal part of your hospital's routine, make sure they provide it for you.

Besides the IV in your arm, you will probably have a **foley catheter** in your bladder that drains urine. The catheter will be removed after twenty-four hours. We are beginning to eliminate this step with select patients. (See box below.)

Outpatient Hip Implant Surgery

The revolution has begun! What once was thought to be impossible is now becoming a reality due to the advances in every aspect of patient care and surgical technique. Recently I did hip implant surgery on a 60-year-old woman. Because she received a minimal dose of anesthesia, she didn't need a foley catheter. The minimal drugs meant she had no nausea. She was able to perform a straight-leg raise immediately after the surgery. She was so stable, she by-passed the recovery room and went straight from the OR to her room where the PTs were waiting to begin gait training.

We have created a team that has modified everything we do: pool prehab to become strong before surgery, minimal drugs, minimally-invasive surgery. As we have improved the safety and the pain control aspect of this procedure, we have made going home the same day after total hip implant surgery a reality. The technology is improving so fast that since we finished the first draft of this book until we worked on final edits, I am now routinely doing this surgery as an outpatient procedure. Select patients are really going home the same day, not to a hotel. We're getting patients back in the game of life so much sooner.

This book gives you everything you need to know to be part of our team.

—Robert Klapper, M.D.

Within a few hours of arriving in your room, you will be getting out of bed. Once the pain is controlled, you will be evaluated by a physical therapist. If you had a regional anesthesia, you must have regained full sensation in both legs. Although you may wish to do nothing but rest, your physical therapists will have specific goals for you even the day of surgery. They will help you sit up on the edge of your bed and dangle your legs over the side. Next they'll help you stand and balance in front of a walker. If it is later in the evening, a nurse rather than a physical therapist will get you up the first time. This might sound a little scary at first, but most patients are thrilled to get up and realize they can put weight on their brand-new hip so soon.

If you managed sitting and standing relatively easily, you'll next be directed to take a few steps on your walker to the nearby chair. Practicing this maneuver from the bed to the chair is called transfer training. You'll sit in the chair briefly, then transfer back into bed. If you don't make it into the chair on the first try, the therapists or nurses will do everything possible to see that you make it on the second try. The success of your surgery will be that much greater the sooner you get going.

By encouraging our patients to do pool therapy prior to surgery, many of them advance quickly on the first day from the walker and crutches to the cane. Some patients feel really good and actually walk with the therapist in the hallway the first day.

Post-Op Days

You will probably be eating regular food by now. The foley catheter will have been removed early in the morning, so when you need to go to the bathroom, you will be assisted by the staff.

It's important to me that I see my patients early the next morning, and I'm hoping your surgeon will do the same. When I make rounds (visits to all my patients in the hospital), I spend time with the patients going over exercises they can do in bed. I explain how important it is for their brains to start talking to their muscles right away. Don't think of this time in bed as being "flat on your back," but rather as time you can use. You've been flexing and pointing your feet. Now you can start gently bending and straightening your knee ever so slightly. Keep trying to move your leg, and soon you'll no longer be afraid of moving it. If you watch TV, do these movements during the commercials, and the repetitions will add up. Then you won't be so wobbly when you stand up to walk because your brain has already been communicating with your muscles.

The physical therapist (PT) will see you in the morning after breakfast and again in the afternoon. They will teach you some basic exercises to strengthen the muscles around your hip. These will be the same exercises they will encourage you to do at home. They will teach you how to get in and out of bed on the same side that you will be using when you return home. Since they like to approximate your bed's height for that practice, it would be good for you to know the distance from the floor to the top of your mattress. The PTs will walk with you down the hallway, sometimes up to two hundred feet. You will probably start on a walker, but as you progress, the PTs may move you from a walker to crutches or to a cane. You will transfer to the chair and be encouraged to sit upright for at least one hour but no more than two hours at a time. If you sit too long too soon, you could easily get stiff.

The nursing staff is trained to help hip implant patients in and out of bed so you do not always need to wait for the therapist. The nurses will encourage you to get out of bed, sit up, and eat your meals. They will remind you to move your ankles up and down, to drink lots of fluids, and to become as independent as possible.

Surgery is premeditated trauma to the body. All the structures that have been addressed—the skin, the muscles, the tendons, and the bones—need time to heal. We know which movements could interrupt the healing at the deep, medium, and surface levels, so specific hip precautions were developed to protect you from making those movements. Those precautions were originally designed to prevent patients from dislocating their new hips. But the risk of dislocation has been greatly reduced in recent years, and many patients will be told they have no movement restrictions. Nevertheless, I'd ask you to consider the big picture following surgery. You have a wound that is very deep—it goes from the skin down to the bone. At the deepest level, your hip joint, once like a lightbulb screwed into a socket, is now more like a plum resting in a coffee cup. Your body needs six weeks to go through the biological process of rebuilding the joint capsule with scar tissue. As we close the other tissues following surgery, the muscles, tendons, and fascia are overlapped and held together with sutures. However, those sutures are as weak as thread; they aren't worth anything in terms of structural strength. By following the hip precautions until these tissues have fused, you won't be pulling on the repair sites where the sutures hold the tissues together. There will be six weeks of tissue healing. You will get a black-and-blue mark that needs to turn green, then yellow. We have not been able to speed up this part of the healing.

Even the incision site on the surface of your skin needs protection. If you make movements that tug on the skin, it may seep a clear fluid and delay the healing process. Although you can shower right away, to promote the fastest healing you want to keep the wound dry. The nurses will instruct you on how to cover the wound for showering with Tegaderm, a waterproof, premade bandage.

During surgery, I move your hip through extreme ranges of motion so I'm confident it won't dislocate. But, call me old-fashioned—I still ask my patients to follow the precautions below. Even if your doctor says you have no movement precautions after your surgery, you can be more comfortable and not disrupt the formation of good scar tissue by following the precautions *whether you were told you need them or not*. You don't have to reach for full motion right away just because you were told you could.

Hip Precautions

Some surgeons no longer suggest hip precautions. Please discuss this with your surgeon and reread the previous paragraph.

- Avoid hip flexion of more than 90 degrees as in these common examples:
  - Avoid lying or sitting on anything low because you will put your hip at risk when trying to get up. Don't sit on the floor or in a vehicle with a low seat.
  - When in bed, don't reach forward past 90 degrees for a pillow or the covers.
  - Don't bend to pick up something from the floor.
  - If your soap falls in the shower, don't bend to pick it up. Have several extra bars handy or buy a soap-on-a-rope for your six-week recovery.
  - Use a high toilet seat so you won't hyperflex your hip when standing up.
- Don't combine hip flexion with internal rotation as shown in Photo 15-1.
- When standing, don't rotate toward your postsurgical side. That causes internal rotation. See Photo 15-2.
- Don't let your ankle or knee cross the midline of your body.
- Don't stand with your feet turned inward.

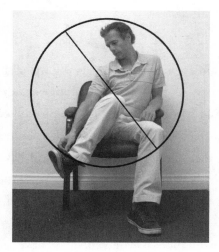

Photo 15-1. Don't combine flexion with internal rotation (assumes the right leg is the surgical leg).

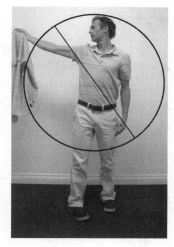

Photo 15-2. Don't rotate toward your postsurgical hip (assumes the right leg is the surgical leg).

Use pain medication if you need it. This isn't the time to turn it down. As your physical therapy becomes more challenging each session, you'll probably need the medication in order to accomplish the tasks that are asked of you. If you say no to pain medication, and then aren't able to do any of the physical therapy because it causes too much pain, you're defeating your recovery program. Ask for painkillers as you need them. As the pain from surgery subsides and you're able to move with less pain, you won't need them as often.

The PT will teach you how to go up and down stairs and how to get in and out of a car (see pages 203 and 204 for specific details). You have a short time to show that you have mastered the basic tasks of living before you can be discharged, so be prepared to be pushed along. However, if you have been moving more slowly than the progress explained here, the demands will be toned down, making it appropriate for you and your current abilities.

The occupational therapist will teach you how to accomplish your tasks of daily living, such as bathing or getting dressed without violating any hip precautions you may have. She'll show you how to use the long-handled devices that help you put on your shoes and socks. Any concerns you have about functioning in your home environment will be discussed, and she'll help you solve those specific details. Nurses will review with you any new medications and their side effects.

Although most patients are discharged on the second day post-op, some patients go home on the first day after surgery.

Going Home

In order to be discharged, you have to have achieved certain goals. The therapists will make sure you can get in and out of bed by yourself and can walk to the bathroom and more than one hundred feet alone, and that you understand the movement precautions so you can be more comfortable. You'll also need to be able to walk up and down however many steps you'll be dealing with at home. If it's time for you to leave the hospital, but you're not doing these things, arrangements will have to be made for you to go to a rehabilitation facility where patients who don't need medical attention can focus on doing intensive physical therapy twice a day while they have someone cooking their meals and caring for them in a nursing setting.

If you live alone, you must be able to perform all of the functions by yourself. If you have someone at home who can help you, you have to be able to do the specified actions with minimal assistance. You'll be evaluated to see whether you meet the criteria for discharge. Assuming you do, your dressing will be changed just before you leave the hospital. You'll leave the dressing on until you visit your surgeon in his or her office, usually a week later.

The nurse or a discharge planner is responsible for coordinating your discharge. He or she can fill your prescriptions prior to discharge, especially pain medication. He or she will also order the equipment you will need and arrange your home physical therapy.

Once you arrive home, a physical therapist or an occupational therapist will visit to see if there are ways to make your home more efficient with your temporary limitations. If this person sees anything of concern, he or she will make adjustments. The goal is to make your home a safe environment.

At Home

You may wonder if you're doing things right or if anything could be going wrong with your hip. Read the box on page 287 for guidance.

Patients ask me all the time what they can do to speed healing. I'm a big believer in taking vitamin C, which is ascorbic acid. Vitamin C is a powerful ingredient in making the bonding glue your body needs to build a healthy scar. When you take increased doses of vitamin C (2000 milligrams per day), it can help your scar heal faster, which accelerates your recovery. Some of you will have to take pills because you have food sensitivities. However, we like to offer holistic options wherever possible, so if you can eat the following foods, you can get your vitamin C naturally. You can create vitamin C-rich juices using oranges, grapefruits, kiwis, tomatoes, and strawberries. But if you can eat red bell peppers, that will be your number-one source of vitamin C in your diet. You or your surgeon may have other ideas regarding diet and nutritional supplements that will best help you heal and stay healthy.

Two weeks later, you'll return to your doctor to have your wound checked. At that same time, seek approval to begin a pool program. You don't have to wait six weeks to start. I'm comfortable letting my patients go into the pool about four weeks after surgery. In the water, you'll be able to perform many safe movements that are still difficult on land. The sooner you start moving, the sooner you'll gain strength to make those same movements against gravity's force on land.

> ### *Driving after Surgery*
>
> How long before you can drive again depends on which hip had the surgery and on what kind of car you drive. If it was your left hip and the car you drive is not too low to the ground or too high and has an automatic shift, you'll be driving a lot sooner than if you had the operation on your right hip and you drive a sports car. It takes longer to feel comfortable driving a stick shift.

Recovery Timeline

Every patient's recovery from surgery is unique. It's hard to give exact times for recovery because much depends on how you answer these questions: How is your general medical health? What is the condition of your other hip? Your back? Your knees? Was there a leg-length problem? Each patient is different, but you will probably return to most, if not all, of your favorite activities. Here are some of the guidelines I suggest to my patients. Discuss your specific case with your surgeon.

- **One to two weeks.** Return to your surgeon to check on your wound healing.
- **Two to six weeks.** It's not a race. You can use a walker, crutches, a cane, or nothing. You'll proceed faster if you did a few months of pool prehab before the surgery. If you didn't train for surgery, or if your back or your other hip hurts, you'll proceed more slowly. But nature still has to run its course, and your wound has to heal. We haven't been able to speed up the six-week healing process. However, the smaller incisions these days let you do basic movements without feeling as wounded and restricted as you would have with the previous implant surgeries.
- **Four Weeks.** As soon as the wound is super-sealed, you can get into the pool.

> ### Brownies Need to Cook for Forty Minutes
>
> The instructions on the box say to cook the brownies for forty minutes. Sure, they start to smell great after twenty minutes. But don't take them out of the oven yet. Leave them in to cook for the full forty minutes. They won't be ready to eat until then.
>
> Consider the "magic number" of six weeks in orthopedics. It takes six weeks for strong tissue healing. Don't start doing inappropriate activities too soon.
>
> —Robert Klapper, MD

- **Six to eight weeks.** You can generally play golf by now.
- **Three months.** You should be at the point where most of the pain from surgery is waning. You may have a morning when you wake up and don't think of your hip as your first thought of the day.
- **Six months.** By now you're far away from the surgery in many ways. You're feeling good about being able to participate in your normal activities.
- **One-year anniversary.** In most cases, this is what your hip is going to be like from now on. The biological remodeling process should be complete, so there aren't likely to be many changes anymore. The scar tissue has evolved: it has healed, broken down, and healed again, finally making functional scar tissue that allows you to move well.
- **Lifetime.** Your new hip needs to be watched, even when it's working well for you. Your surgeon will most likely want you to come for regular checkups every few years. Over 90 percent of the patients with hip implants are still doing well fifteen or twenty years later, and we expect some of the newer implants we're using to last up to thirty years. Just how long any implant will last depends on the bone, the implant, and the patient.

You elected to undergo implant surgery for various reasons: to return to your athletic or sexual activities, to sleep without pain through the night, or to be able to walk well again, among other concerns. Disability in a hip joint causes possibly the most severe life limitations of all joint dysfunctions. When you're able to return to your normal life with a hip joint that functions fully without pain, your days will feel like a legitimate miracle. The implant will make a huge difference in the quality of your life. If you decide to choose this option, it's a significant undertaking, but one with great rewards. Of all the surgical procedures studied by researchers, the highest satisfaction rate comes from hip implant patients.

Your life will be returned to you to enjoy.

16

AFTER SURGERY: REHAB PROGRAMS

Memory can be your worst enemy in the weeks and months following surgery. You remember how far you used to run or walk, how many sets of tennis you used to play, or how many golf courses you used to visit each year. You will probably find that "used to" phrase in both your thoughts and your conversations. But as basketball legend Wilt Chamberlain always said, "Old Man 'Used To' is dead and gone." What you used to do no longer applies. Forget it, and start where you are right now.

Your postsurgical hip requires planning, pampering, and patience. You need to plan your recovery with care, pamper your aching hip that sometimes won't feel as if it belongs to you, and have patience knowing that the human body heals. That's what it is programmed to do. "Tincture of Time" plus ice and the proper exercises will help you regain your strength and flexibility. Soon enough you will be mobile and comfortable as you move through your daily life and recreational activities.

Every patient's recovery from surgery is different. Much depends on your general medical health, your presurgery fitness level, your age, and the condition of your other hip, your knees, and your back. Still, you will probably return to most if not all of your favorite activities. We will offer guidelines for safely progressing through your recovery, but you should discuss your specific case with your surgeon.

You may have already learned the exercises in the pool and land programs in chapters 9 and 12 as you tried to prevent hip surgery. Your efforts may have turned into prehab, which is rehabilitation prior to surgery. In that case, you entered the operating room stronger and fitter because you prepared for the rigors of surgery. Some of you may have found this book only after you had hip surgery and now you intend to use our pool and land programs to speed your recovery.

Our protocol for recovery from implant surgery has a long track record of success. However, since we're still in the evolutionary stage of arthroscopic surgeries for FAI and labral repair, the surgical techniques as well as the ideas for rehabilitation are still evolving. We worked with hip arthroscopist Jason Snibbe, MD, to develop the pool and land protocol for arthroscopy that starts on page 296. **But you must also consult with your own surgeon.**

Three Phases of Postsurgical Rehabilitation

As you learn about the three phases of healing, your recovery will begin to make sense. You can set your sights on specific milestones rather than on your temporary disability. You won't feel like the only person who ever had this pain or ache or experienced what you are going through.

The three phases of recovery are defined not by specific timelines, but rather by a decrease in symptoms, an increase in function, and an ability to return to your previous activities. Because each individual has different healing times, some will progress faster than others. For this reason hip implant patients do not have specific time frames for recovery and should not feel discouraged if their recovery is taking longer than someone else's. In comparison, hip arthroscopy patients have strict precautions that initially follow a timeline due to the intricate surgical work performed inside the hip joint.

Phase One

Right after surgery, you will find yourself in the first phase of rehabilitation, which is characterized by the following:

Pain. The body's pain receptors are sensitive to hot and cold, vibration, stretch, and inflammation. You will have nearly constant moderate to severe pain every day. You may even begin to notice increased pain in your nonsurgical leg due to the extra work it is doing.

Inflammation. The signs of inflammation are pain, heat, redness, swelling, and loss of function. Inflammation is a protective attempt by the body to start the healing process and remove the damaging stimulus.

Swelling. Swelling is the body's natural response to trauma in order to immobilize the area. Because swelling immobilizes the injured area, it causes a loss of movement. At the same time, it causes increased pain as it puts pressure on the nerves.

Loss of mobility. Swelling causes increased pressure within your hip joint and the surrounding tissues, which makes it difficult to move your hip. Your pain also stimulates "splinting," or increased muscular contraction around the area to further immobilize and protect your hip.

Loss of function. When you lose mobility in your hip, you also lose function. When the muscles are in "splinting" mode, your hip can quickly become stiff. You will likely notice difficulty with standing up from a chair or getting in and out of a car.

Rapid loss of fitness level. Anyone who has been physically active will tell you how fast he or she gets out of shape after an injury. Now, without mobility and function in your hip, you will lose fitness. Unless you quickly begin rehabilitation exercises, your overall body fitness will quickly decline. Specifically, the muscle strength of your postsurgical leg will weaken unless you start using it right away.

The goals of Phase One are to resolve all the above issues, but the major emphasis is on eliminating pain, inflammation, and swelling. All six of the above factors are easily addressed in the pool. The cooling effect of the water helps decrease pain and inflammation while the hydrostatic pressure the water exerts on your body helps push out swelling. You will be able to move much sooner and more easily in water than you can on land, so begin your postsurgical rehab as soon as your doctor tells you your incision site is healed enough and you've been approved to get into the pool.

You'll begin land exercises right away as well. If an exercise increases your hip pain, skip it and try the next exercise. If the land exercises seem too difficult or painful at first, start your rehab in the pool. If you don't have access to a pool, you'll focus on the land exercises as soon as you are able.

You'll be surprised how quickly you can bear weight on your affected leg. Most postsurgical hip patients are up and walking on their new hips the day of surgery or the day after. You may need a walker, crutches, or a cane, but work on normalizing your walking pattern right away to avoid developing bad habits. Don't be too proud to use these devices. They are an important part of the recovery of even the world's best athletes. If you have any restrictions on weight bearing, your surgeon will give them to you.

Phase Two

You enter Phase Two when you can identify your first significant reduction of symptoms. This means you have less pain and swelling as well as improved mobility and function. In Phase Two you have mild to moderate intermittent pain that comes from movement related to your activities of daily living. Although your symptoms have begun to decrease, moderate inflammation and swelling are still present and a moderate loss of mobility and function still exists. Nevertheless, it is time to begin regaining strength and flexibility to prepare for the more strenuous rehabilitation to come. You can expect to feel some mild to moderate pain when you move your hip, but don't force an exercise or increase your pain beyond that moderate level.

Your goals in Phase Two continue to be the reduction of pain, inflammation, and swelling; however, the major emphasis turns to increasing your flexibility and strength so you can return to normal weight bearing and walking.

Phase Three

Phase Three begins when you can accomplish basic movement around the house and can perform common everyday activities. Your pain should be mild and occur only during movement. Inflammation and swelling will be minimal. You may not have mastered higher-level activities such as recreational sports or sitting down without using your arms. It is during Phase Three that many people stop short of their goals for full recovery. The almost-imperceptible swelling, chronic inflammation, incomplete range of motion, and decrease in strength are the last traces of your surgery, and they are very real obstacles to regaining full function.

Keep going with your pool and land rehabilitation exercises until you reach the goals of Phase Three: to be relatively pain-free with few or no symptoms. Before you're finished, you want to be free of all swelling and inflammation and should have full strength and range of motion. These goals may take up to a year to accomplish. *The higher the expectations you have for your hip and its long-term function, the longer you'll need to continue your rehabilitation.* Follow the detailed pool and land therapy protocols for hip arthroscopy and for hip implant surgery on the following pages.

Phase Three is where this program can help you the most. You will probably have an experienced physical therapist help you through the first few difficult months. But the biological remodeling inside your hip joint takes up to a year, as can regaining your full strength. All you need is to make time in your schedule and use the instructions in this book as your exercise program. You can make the strength phase be the most self-propelled.

Remain Cautious and Deliberate

Somewhere in the middle of a rehab session, when you're doing exceptionally well, you may have the thought, *I could go surfing*, or *I could play tennis—today!* **Don't.** Continue to be cautious and deliberate throughout your rehab period, and your progress will generally be steady and consistent. If you do too much too quickly, you can cause a setback that brings pain, swelling, and undue soreness. That may mean you have to spend extra days in the pool away from gravity. Don't get upset. Vow not to make the same mistake that triggered the setback, and do the pool recovery work to get back to where you were. By assuming full responsibility for your hip and any risks you take with it, you can earn a hip that serves you beautifully for a lifetime.

—Lynda Huey

If you had arthroscopic hip surgery, continue reading the next section, where you'll find your three phases of rehabilitation. If you had hip implant surgery, follow the program that begins on page 306. Others who don't fall cleanly into one of these categories can still use these programs. There are a great variety of fractures that can happen to the femur, the pelvis, and the pelvic area. Your surgeon will determine how much healing time you require before beginning pool therapy and if there are specific weight-bearing and movement precautions to follow. Some fractures that are more stable can tolerate pool therapy much sooner than others that are more critical in their location. *This decision must be made by your orthopedic surgeon.* For all fractures of the pelvis and femur, use the implant protocol that starts on page 306.

Arthroscopic Surgery

Since arthroscopic surgeries use only small puncture incisions to enter your hip joint, they are considered minimally invasive. But they still require extra caution for the first few months because extensive work is performed inside the joint. Bone has been remodeled for those with FAI, and sutures or grafts have been anchored to the bone for labral reconstructions.

These are our suggestions, but you should speak to your own surgeon before beginning any exercise program. He or she is the one who saw inside your joint and knows what work was done that needs protecting. He or she may offer a different series of exercises.

Our pool program does not require that you know how to swim, but swimmers often ask us if they can swim through their recovery. Swimming maximizes the recovery of the hip because it's such a gluteal-based exercise, but note the limitation of no kicking until the six-week mark below. A stationary bike is good to increase range of motion and prevent **adhesions**, but strengthening of the gluteals is better in the pool. See details in the pool and land program on the following pages.

Phase One

Your wound is healing for the first few weeks. The internal repairs your surgeon made will be healing for the first six weeks, which means you'll wait to move to Phase Two until six weeks after surgery. Focus on starting the process of regaining your range of motion as well as establishing a normalized gait (walking pattern).

You can ride a stationary bike the day after surgery, starting at five minutes twice a day with minimal resistance. You can also take a short walk three times a day as tolerated. But that's it. The first week is the time to let your hip calm down. Walk and bike to activate your muscles, and keep icing.

Ask your surgeon if he or she will allow you to do the Snibbe Stretch, Exercise 5 on page 214. Dr.

Snibbe tells his patients they can start doing this stretch one week after surgery, and as the weeks go by, they can lift the knee higher and push harder into the stretch. At six weeks he lets patients push even harder into the stretch three times a day. He expects them to do this stretch throughout their entire recovery. *But speak with your own surgeon to get approval.*

Once you've been approved to enter the pool, put your focus there. If you've been frustrated from lack of movement, you will greatly enjoy your first day in the pool. You'll leave gravity behind and move easily and comfortably as you start your rehab.

If you have been working out regularly prior to surgery, you can go to the pool every day as long as you don't have any adverse effects or increased pain. If you were not in good shape prior to surgery, skip a day between sessions your first week or two, and concentrate on icing your hip on your off days. When you begin the land program, notice whether you feel an increase in pain, inflammation, or swelling after the session. If so, stick with the pool for another post-op week.

Get the Most from Your Postsurgical Sessions

Ice after each session. Ice can make the difference between recovering well from a session or not. If you ice immediately afterward, you may not be sore, stiff, or have as much pain the next day.

Don't try to do too much. You'll know you worked too hard if pain and swelling increase after the session and persist even after you ice. Sometimes you can sleep that off, but if pain and swelling persist more than twenty-four hours, cut back your workout intensity by reducing your reps and moving more slowly.

Do *only* the Phase One exercises when you're in Phase One. Stick with the phase you're really in—don't jump around out of curiosity or optimism. When you meet all the criteria for moving to the next phase, you can then increase your exercises per the protocols to follow.

Begin slowly, move gently, and proceed with caution. If you feel increased pain, narrow your range of motion or move even more slowly. Follow this Phase One program until your symptoms begin to subside.

POOL:

Start slowly and proceed with caution. The water will feel so liberating that you might be tempted to test your hip by moving it through its entire range of motion the moment you step into the pool. Your enthusiasm is a great sign, but restrain yourself! Follow whatever restrictions your surgeon has given you. Remember that you most likely have healing bone and sutures inside the joint, so be cautious as you begin, and remain vigilant throughout your first six weeks. And yet you have only the first six weeks after surgery to regain your internal rotation. If you don't work on it in the beginning, you won't get it back. You must walk a fine line between caution and reaching for increased internal rotation as you do Exercise 6.1 on page 179. Do it gently, but do it diligently every time you're in the pool.

To protect your healing hip from impact, put on your flotation belt and do the non-weight-bearing, Deep-Water Exercises that begin on page 143. (See pages 117 to 119 for help in selecting the correct flotation belt for your body type.) If you're a non-swimmer, you can hold the side of the pool while you do the poolside variations of these exercises as shown on page 133. You don't have to go into a corner as shown if that seems too far away. Move just deep enough in the pool that your feet do not touch the pool bottom. That's far enough! Now hold on and start the Running, Walking, and Flies without any weight bearing, and you'll soon agree it's worth finding the courage to stay right there for the fifteen minutes it takes to do your deep-water intervals. Most of the other kicks and exercises can be performed in the shallow end of the pool. Follow your surgeon's advice whether you should cross your legs or not on Scissors in the Kicking Series, and work your way from ten reps to twenty reps on the Lower Body Exercises by adding two reps each pool session.

If You Don't Have Deep Water

If you don't have access to deep water, face the side of the pool and lean forward for running with your feet pushing down at an angle behind you, not touching the pool bottom. For Power Walk and Flies, turn your back to the side of the pool, and let your hips float up about halfway toward the surface as you move your legs against the water's resistance. Avoid impact with the pool bottom and thus prevent weight bearing.

- **Gait Training:** Walking Forward, Backward, Sideways   2 minutes each walk
  (See Exercise 1 page 129.
- **Deep-Water Intervals:** low-intensity level   15 minutes total
  (See Exercises 4–6, pages 132 to 135 and Exercise 8, page 136.)
- **Stretching:** Hamstring Stretch, Quad Stretch, Hip Flexor Stretch   30 seconds each
  (See Exercises 9, 12, and 13, pages 140 and 142.)
- **Kicking Series:** Bicycling, Deep Back Kick, Straight-Leg Deep Kick,
  Scissors, crossing or no crossing   30 seconds each
  (See Exercises 18–21, pages 147 to 150.)
- **Lower Body Exercises:** Lateral Leg Raises, Leg Circles, Knee Swivels,
  Two-Way Hip   10 to 20 reps each
  (See Exercises 35, 37–38, and 40, pages 163, 164 to 166 and 169 to 170.)
  (See appendix to order equipment.)

LAND:

During your first week after surgery, you will limit yourself to icing, walking, and stationary biking. Starting the second week, you'll perform Stretching and Internal Rotation only. *Exercise 5, Snibbe Stretch, should be done at least three times a day to stretch your joint capsule.*

Observe the warnings in chapter 12 that ask you to get your surgeon's approval before starting certain exercises. Stay within your pain-free range of motion, which is especially important while you're healing after surgery. Let pain be your guide. Move your hip only to the point where you feel some discomfort. Do not create more pain. Begin by doing each of the stretches three times for thirty seconds (except Snibbe Stretch, which is held for up to two minutes). Ice after each session with your leg elevated. You may be surprised how easily you will be walking in just a week. By starting these land exercises right away, you'll increase the blood flow and strengthen the muscles needed to perform your daily functional activities.

You need to work on your internal rotation in the first six weeks or you may never regain it. So you'll do Exercise 17, Internal Rotation, but without the Thera-Band. Start with ten repetitions and work your way up to twenty reps during Phase 1. In Phase Two, you'll add the Thera-Band.

- **Stretching**: Hamstring Stretch, Knee to Chest Stretch,
  Hip Extensor Stretch, Snibbe Stretch (up to 2 minutes},
  Prone Quad Stretch
  (See Exercises 1-3 and 5-6, pages 210 to 212 and 214 to 215.)   3 x 30 seconds (except Snibbe)
- **Internal Rotation**:
  Exercise 17, no Thera-Band   10 to 20 reps
- **Bicycling**: Stationary or recumbent bike   5 to 10 minutes,
                                                                         minimum resistance

Some surgeons will say you must wait until the six-week mark to do the Basic Exercises; others will say you can begin sooner. Notice that we eliminated Straight Leg Raises and Clamshells for our hip arthroscopy patients since those exercises may trigger hip flexor tendinitis. Ask your surgeon when and if you can do the Basic Exercises listed here:

- **Basic Exercises**: Prone Hip Extension, Ball Squeeze with   10 reps
  Abdominal Contraction, Bridge, Hip Extension
  (See Exercises 7,9-10, and 13, pages 216, 218 and 220.}

Phase Two

Your internal surgical repairs have mended by the six-week mark, so that's when Phase Two will begin. Your pain, inflammation, and swelling normally have come down now. It's time to increase your workload by adding more exercises, more sets, and more repetitions (reps). Although you started gentle range of motion exercises in Phase One, now is the time to achieve greater range of motion on your surgical side. Here's where a physical therapist is of great value. The hands-on guidance they offer is reassuring when you may not quite know the correct effort level to use.

Notice how both your pool and land programs have nearly doubled in length. This is where you will begin to feel yourself getting stronger and more capable in your daily life. You may even be starting to daydream about your sports life as well.

POOL:

You have been doing exercises that are great for regaining gluteal strength and for re-educating your gluteal muscles on how and when to fire in the proper sequence. They are: Exercise 5, Power Walk; Exercise 19, Deep Back Kick; and Exercise 40, Two-Way Hip. Now it's time to test out Exercise 7, Speed Walk, to see if your hip is ready to begin working your hip flexors and gluteals alternatingly in rapid-fire succession. If this challenging exercise hurts your hip, or if you experience increased pain for more than twenty-four hours after doing it, wait another few weeks before trying to add it to your program again.

You'll also be adding your first exercises that call for low impact in the shallow end of the pool, so notice that you **must** wear a flotation belt in this phase. Read the introduction to Impact Exercises on pages 151 to 152 in chapter 9, then the material specific to postsurgical patients on page 189 in chapter 10. There you should find the reassurance and courage you need to try these enjoyable exercises. Start with the First Four exercises only, as explained on page 151. If you feel good the next day at the pool, you can start adding other Impact Exercises as suggested.

If you're a runner, get ready! Nothing is as satisfying as running with your feet on the bottom of the pool. Your arms push hard against the water in opposition to your legs, and for brief moments, you'll be able to picture yourself back in your running life. This alone may be what brings you back time and again to the pool. Keep your float belt on as you begin Exercise 34, Shallow-Water Running in chest-deep water.

- **Gait Training:** All

  (See Exercises 1–3, pages 129 to 131.)   1 minute each walk

- **Deep-Water Intervals:** All, medium-intensity level   20 minutes total

  (See Exercises 4–8, pages 132 to 136.)

- **Stretching:** All   1 minute each

  (See Exercises 9–13, pages 140 to 142.)

- **Kicking Series:** All   45 seconds each

  (See Exercises 17–21, pages 146 to 150.)

- **Impact Exercises:**   10 reps <u>with belt</u>

  Lunges, Jacks, Squat Jumps, Power Frogs (First Four)   progress to 20 reps

  (See Exercises 22–25, pages 152 to 154.)

  Add a few more Impact Exercises each session.

  Running <u>with belt</u>, low-intensity program   2 to 6 minutes

  (See Exercise 34, page 160.)

- **Lower Extremity Exercises:** As appropriate per warnings   20 reps each

  (See Exercises 35–38, pages 163 to 166.)

  Add Aqualogix blade, minimum resistance   progress to maximum resistance

LAND:

If your surgeon told you to skip the Basic Exercises for six weeks, you'll start doing them now, one set of ten reps. If you started them in Phase One, increase your number of Basic Exercise repetitions to two sets of ten reps, or twenty reps total.

If you're able to stand on your surgical leg for three to five seconds without any instability, you'll also start to add the Resistance, Stability Ball, Balance, and Functional Exercises in Phase Two. When you do Exercises 14–17, begin with no resistance, then progress to the easiest (yellow) Thera-band. Increase to a stronger Thera-Band each week if you can comfortably perform your repetitions. If you feel fatigued after ten reps, stay with that same color Thera-Band until the ten reps become easy. (See chart on page 220 for color progression of Thera-Bands.)

- **Stretching:** Hamstring Stretch, Knee to Chest Stretch, Hip Extensor Stretch, Snibbe Stretch (up to 2 minutes), Prone Quad Stretch
(See Exercises 1–3 and 5–6, pages 210 to 212 and 214 to 215.)

  3 x 30 seconds (except Snibbe)

- **Basic Exercises:** Prone Hip Extension, Ball Squeeze with Abdominal Contraction, Bridges, Side-Lying Hip Abduction, Hip Extension,
(See Exercises 7, 9–11, and 13, pages 216, 218 to 219 and 220.)

  10 reps (if first time)
  2 x 10 reps (if 10 reps in phase one)

- **Resistance Exercises:** Hip Extension with Thera-Band, Hip Abduction with Thera-Band, Hip External Rotation with Thera-Band, Hip Internal Rotation with Thera-Band
(See Exercises 14–17, pages 221 to 224.)

  10 reps

  10 reps

- **Stability Ball Exercises:** Bridge on Ball, Bridge on Ball with Leg Lift, Bridge on Ball with Hamstring Curl
(See Exercises 18–20, pages 226 to 227.)

  10 reps

- **Balance Exercises:** Single Leg Balance, Clocks with Single Leg Balance, Hamstring Curls
(See Exercises 21–23, pages 228 to 230.)

  2 X 30 seconds

- **Functional Exercises:** Sit to Stand, Step Over and Back
(See Exercises 24–25, pages 231 to 232.)

  10 reps

- **Bicycling:** Stationary or recumbent bike

  10-20 minutes
  moderate tension

Phase Three

Now you're ready for increased impact in the pool and more repetitions of the functional exercises on land. You're running and jumping in the pool by now, so notice that gait training is no longer in your program. In Phase Two, you did the four safest Impact Exercises while wearing a flotation belt. You jumped upward using your muscular strength, but the belt, not your hip, caught most of your weight as you landed. If you added all the Impact Exercises to your program in Phase Two, you may now remove the flotation belt. If you were doing twenty reps, cut back to fifteen reps the first session. You'll be surprised how much harder the exercises are without your belt, so don't try for too many reps too quickly. You can move up to twenty reps again the next week. Similarly, when you add resistance pieces to your lower extremity exercises, you'll feel how much harder the exercise is, so drop your reps from twenty to fifteen, and work your way back up over the next few sessions. Then move up to the next higher resistance piece. This may seem slow, but it's your surest way to progress without re-injury. There are two levels of Aqualogix Blades—low and high resistance. The Hydro-Tone Boot is the highest of all resistance. Not everyone will progress to that piece or even like it. Stick with the one that feels challenging but comfortable to you. Use it from now on.

If you had a labral reconstruction, patiently focus on gluteal strengthening for extra weeks or even months. Unless you work diligently to regain the balance of strength between your gluteal and hip flexor muscles, you could create a nasty case of hip flexor tendinitis for yourself. But even if you do start getting hip flexor pain around the three-month mark, don't be discouraged. It's a normal thing to feel. Keep strengthening your gluteal muscles and around the six-month mark, you should feel that you've broken through that problem, and you'll be happy.

In your land program, you'll increase your reps by one set. You'll continue to progress to more difficult Thera-Bands as you do your resistance exercises. Begin Phase Three with the Thera-Band color that allows you to comfortably perform eight repetitions but feel fatigued after ten reps. See the table on page 220 in chapter 12 that shows the progression in Thera-Band colors.

You will have very few restrictions if you've had a normal recovery. If you've had difficulties, make sure you have a conversation with your surgeon before you add new exercises such as the Deep-Water Exercises 14 to 16.

POOL:

- **Deep-Water Intervals:** high-intensity level   25 minutes total
  (See Exercises 4–8, pages 132 to 136.)
- **Stretching:** All   1 minute each
  (See Exercises 9–13, pages 140 to 142.)
- **Deep-Water Exercises:** All   30 reps each
  (See Exercises 14–16, pages 143 to 144.)
- **Kicking Series:** All   1 minute each
  (See Exercises 17–21, pages 146 to 150.
  Work harder the last 30 seconds.)

- **Impact Exercises:** All (no belt)   20 reps, jump higher on the last 10

  (See Exercises 22–33, pages 152 to 159.

  When belt is removed, start at 15 reps again.

  Work back up to 20 reps.)

  Running, no belt, high-intensity program   5-10 minutes

  (See Exercise 34, page 160.)

- **Lower Extremity Exercises:** As appropriate per warnings   20 reps each

  Add increased resistance equipment,

  (See Exercises 35–38, and Exercise 40, pages 163 to 166

  and pages 169 to 170.)

LAND:

- **Stretching:** Hamstring Stretch, Knee to Chest Stretch,   3 x 30 seconds (except Snibbe)

  Hip Extensor Stretch, Iliotibial Band Stretch,

  Snibbe Stretch (up to two minutes), Prone Quad Stretch

  (See Exercises 1–6, page 210 to 215.)

- **Basic Exercises:** Prone Hip Extension, Ball Squeeze   2 x 10 reps

  with Abdominal Contraction, Bridges, Side-Lying

  Hip Abduction, Hip Extension,

  (See Exercises 7, 9–11, and 13, pages 216 and 218 to 220)

- **Resistance Exercises:** All   2 x 10 reps

  (See Exercises 14–17, pages 221 to 224.)

- **Stability Ball Exercises:** All   2 x 10 reps

  (See Exercises 18–20, pages 226 to 227.)

- **Balance Exercises:** All   3 x 30 seconds

  (See Exercises 21–23 on pages 228 to 230.)

- **Functional Exercises:** All   2 x 10 reps

  (See Exercises 24–25, pages 231 to 232.)

- **Bicycling:** Stationary or recumbent bike   20-30 minutes moderate tension

Hip Implant Surgery

Hip implant patients recover more fully than any of the other joint replacement patients. It may feel like a big surgery—and it is. But it will be forever worth the recovery time once your new hip is rolling along at full speed. The constant bone-on-bone pain you had in your hip will be gone after surgery, and you can look forward to regaining all of the movement you had before your hip became problematic. Of course you have to get through the postsurgical pain you currently have, which is what Phase One is all about.

You are going to be thrilled when you get into the pool, and the buoyancy of the water lifts your leg through a wider range of motion than you could have imagined with your old hip. You may feel like showing off how much better and farther this new hip can move, but remember to be cautious, start slowly, and move gently at first. All the tissues that were cut from the skin down deep to the joint must heal. There's no way around it—that's going to take six weeks. If your surgeon gave you hip precautions, follow the limited versions of the exercises where suggested. Many surgeons have new techniques that no longer require such limitations, but if your surgeon told you specific hip precautions, honor them! (You can read the most common precautions on page 284.) Our suggestion is a middle ground: even if you weren't given any movement restrictions following surgery, you don't have to reach for full motion right away. By at least paying lip service to the precautions, you can be a lot more comfortable for the first six weeks and at the same time not disrupt tissue healing.

Phase One

When you go home, you will be on crutches or a walker. Older patients will use a walker and then progress to a cane. Younger patients will most likely use crutches. While you can expect soreness, swelling, and heat, be aware of any sudden changes in the appearance of your incision. (See page 287 regarding postsurgical emergencies.)

The emphasis during the first four weeks is on controlling swelling and pain. Since you may not be allowed into the pool for four weeks, you'll be recovering with land treatments such as ice, stretches, and some basic exercises. Once you're in the water, you'll start with gait training, which consists of walking while focusing on good form. This is a great way to reteach yourself to walk without a limp.

Don't be surprised if you progress quickly, both on land and in the pool. Notice that you'll be doing a good number of stretches and exercises even here in Phase One. In the pool, you'll add a mini buoyancy cuff by about your third visit, which will help you improve your range of motion. When that gets easy, move to the standard buoyancy cuff. You'll feel about three times as much lift from that larger piece. If it's too much, go back to the mini cuff for another week or two.

POOL:

During your first week in the water, do only the pain-free exercises. That means if an exercise hurts, you should skip it. You can also do less time and fewer reps than what is listed if the program seems too difficult. By the second week, however, start doing all the exercises, even if very slowly. If you experience pain, slow the movement or narrow the range of motion. If your hip is stiff or swollen, gently try to loosen it by slowly continuing the exercise with care. The pool exercises will help improve your circulation, and the hydrostatic pressure will help push out the fluids of swelling. The Hip Flexor Stretch may be hard for you to do. You can put a strap around your foot and pull it over your shoulder to manually assist yourself into the position.

- **Gait Training:** Walking Forward, Backward, Sideways, Marching
  (See Exercises 1–2, page 129 and 130.) — 2 minutes each walk

- **Deep-Water Intervals:** low-intensity level
  (See Exercises 4–6 and 8, pages 132 to 135 and 136.) — 15 minutes total

- **Stretching:** Hamstring Stretch, Body Swing, Lateral Stretch
  (See Exercises 9–11, pages 140 to 141.) — 30 seconds each

- **Kicking Series:** All kicks within precautions
  (See Exercises 17–21, pages 146 to 150.) — 30 seconds each

- **Lower Body Exercises:** Lateral Leg Raises, Leg Swings, Leg Circles both directions, Knee Swivels
  (See Exercises 35–38, pages 163 to 166.) — 15 reps each
  Add mini buoyancy cuff by third visit, progress to standard cuff

LAND:

Your land program will begin in the second week. You'll get started on basic strengthening through your activities of daily living (ADLs). Probably the most important activity of life is being able to walk from one place to another. You'll want to work on creating a normal gait (walking pattern) both in the pool and on land. Establish good walking form in the pool, then try it against gravity on land. Make note of any difficulties you're having, and work on them again the next time you're in the pool. Think of the pool as the learning site, where your body doesn't have to combat gravity. You can focus on good form without carrying all your weight. On land, you have to shift your weight as you balance rather than let the water hold you up. Pool/land/pool/land is the perfect combination. Keep trying until your therapist, coach, or training partner tells you that you're walking well.

- **Stretching:** Hamstring Stretch, Knee to Chest Stretch, Hip Extensor Stretch, Snibbe Stretch (up to 2 minutes), Prone Quad Stretch
(See Exercises 1–3, and 5–6, pages 210 to 212 and 214 to 215.)
  — 3 x 30 seconds (except Snibbe)

- **Basic Exercises:** Prone Hip Extension, Straight Leg Raise, Ball Squeeze with Abdominal Contraction, Bridges, Clamshells, Hip Extension
(See Exercises 7–10 and 12–13, pages 216 to 220.)
  — 10 reps

- **Resistance Exercises:** Hip Abduction, no Thera-Band
(See Exercise 15, page 222.)
  — 10 reps

- **Functional Exercises:** Sit to Stand
(See Exercise 24, page 231.)
  — 10 reps

  Bicycling: Stationary or recumbent bike
  — 5-10 minutes with zero resistance

Phase Two

In Phase Two your pain won't be as constant or as intense. Your range of motion will begin to improve so you'll be able to perform your activities of daily living more easily. It won't be as difficult to rise from a toilet or a chair, your hip won't feel as stiff when walking, and you may be able to climb stairs leading with your surgical leg. Descending stairs may still be difficult, but don't worry—that's normal. Hold the railing as you practice, and you'll keep getting better at it, especially if you focus on doing stair work regularly and with good form. Remember that you are still healing, so don't overdo any activities. If your surgeon allows, you may be able to start doing some light exercise on an elliptical machine.

In the pool, you'll add Exercise 7, Speed Walk, to your Deep-Water Intervals. This exercise will help you build core, gluteal, and thigh strength while you also fine-tune your coordination. At this stage, the Hip Flexor Stretch may be hard for you to do. You can put a strap around your foot and pull it over your shoulder to manually assist yourself into the position. You'll do the First Four Impact Exercises **while wearing a flotation belt.** Read the section in chapter 9 on how to ease into the Impact Exercises with the proper gradients of increased weight bearing on page 151 to 152.

POOL:

- **Gait Training:** All   1 minute each walk
  (See Exercises 1–3, pages 129 to 131.)
- **Deep-Water intervals:** medium-intensity level   20 minutes total
  (See Exercises 4–8, pages 132 to 136.)
- **Stretching:** All   1 minute each
  (See Exercises 9–13, pages 140 to 142.)
  Quad Stretch and Hip Flexor Stretch with strap or
  assistance
- **Kicking Series:** All   45 seconds each
  (See Exercises 17–21, pages 146 to 150.)
- **Impact Exercises:** First Four, add more each visit   10 to 20 reps <u>with belt</u>
  (See Exercises 22–25, pages 152 to 154.)
  Add Exercises 26–33, pages 154 to 159 over a few weeks
  Running, <u>with belt</u>, low- to moderate-intensity program   2 to 10 minutes
  (See Exercise 34 on page 160.)

- **Lower Body Exercises:** All   20 reps each
  (See Exercises 35–39, pages 163 to 168.)
  Switch from buoyancy cuff to low-resistance blade,
  progress to high-resistance blade.

LAND:

- **Stretching:** Hamstring Stretch, Knee to Chest Stretch,   3 x 30 seconds (except Snibbe)
  Hip Extensor Stretch, Snibbe Stretch (up to 2 minutes),
  Prone Quad Stretch
  (See Exercises 1–3, 5–6, pages 210 to 212 and 214 to 215.)
- **Basic Exercises:** All   20 reps
  (See Exercises 7–13, pages 216 to 220.)
- **Resistance Exercises:** All   10 reps
  (See Exercises 14–17, pages 221 to 224.)
- **Stability Ball Exercises:** All   10 reps
  (See Exercises 18–20, pages 226 to 227.)
- **Balance Exercises:** All   2 x 30 seconds
  (See Exercises 21–23, pages 228 to 230.)
- **Functional Exercises:** All   10 reps
  (See Exercises 24–25, page 231 to 232.)
- **Bicycling:** Stationary or recumbent bike   10 to 20 minutes with
  moderate tension

Phase Three

A lot of healing has occurred, and you're able to do much more by now. You are most likely performing your daily life activities without discomfort. You may still be experiencing stiffness, but your pain will be minimal and subsiding. During Phase Three you'll find you can accomplish more challenging functional activities such as climbing a flight of stairs with a reciprocal pattern, rising from a lower chair, and squatting to a deeper position. Descending stairs may still be difficult. Fine-tuning your normal pattern for climbing stairs will be one of the most challenging of the last goals you'll accomplish.

When doing the Impact Exercises in chest-deep water, you'll increase your intensity and reps and you'll remove your flotation belt—a very big accomplishment. But keep the belt handy as your backup plan, and use it any day you feel pain or discomfort. Just by adding the belt, you'll probably be able to continue with all your Impact Exercises. Enjoy your ability to run and jump with Exercises 22–34.

On land, you'll be doing all of the Functional and Resistance Exercises.

POOL:

- **Gait training:** All   1 minute each
  (See Exercises 1–3, pages 129 to 131.)
- **Deep-Water Intervals:** All, high-intensity level   20 minutes total
  (See Exercises 4–8, pages 132 to 136.)
- **Stretching:** All   1 minute each
  (See Exercises 9–13, pages 140 to 142.)
- **Deep-Water Exercises:** All   20 to 30 reps each
  (See Exercises 14–16, pages 143 to 144.)
- **Kicking Series:** All   1 minute each
  (See Exercises 17–21, pages 146 to 150.)
  Increase speed and effort the last 30 seconds.)
- **Impact Exercises:** All   20 reps, no belt
  (See Exercises 22–33, pages 152 to 159.)
  Running, no belt, moderate- to high-intensity   10 to 15 minutes
  (See Exercise 34, page 160.)
- **Lower Extremity Exercises:** All   20 reps each
  (See Exercises 35–39, pages 163 to 165.)
  Increase resistance.

LAND:

- **Stretching:** All   3 x 30 seconds (except Snibbe)
  (See Exercises 1–6, pages 210 to 215.)

- **Basic Exercises:** All   3 x 30 reps
  (See Exercises 7–13, pages 216 to 220.)

- **Resistance Exercises:** All   20 reps
  (See Exercises 14–17, pages 221 to 224.)

- **Stability Ball Exercises:** All   20 reps
  (See Exercises 18–20, pages 226 to 227.)

- **Balance Exercises:** All   3 x 30 seconds
  (See Exercises 21–23, pages 228 to 230.)

- **Functional Exercises:** All   20 reps
  (See Exercises 24–25, pages 231 to 232.)

- **Bicycling:** Stationary or recumbent bike   20 to 30 minutes moderate tension

Your Maintenance Program

You're probably breathing a huge sigh of relief now that you've completed all three phases of your hip rehabilitation. Yet in spite of all the work you've already put into your healing hip, the work cannot stop here. You need to continue exercising for the rest of your life. Don't panic; you don't need to work at the same frequency of five times a week—three to four times a week at the level of your Phase Three program should be fine. If you feel dysfunction creeping into your hip from lack of exercise, you can always resume the full-fledged program. Take charge of your hip; keep it strong and functioning smoothly so it can serve you for many years, hopefully an entire lifetime.

GLOSSARY

abduct to move a body part away from the midline of the body.

abduction movement away from the midline of the body. Applied to the hip, it means moving the leg out to the side.

abusive activities which cause damage to your weight-bearing joints.

acetabulum located in the pelvis, it is the socket side of the hip's ball-and-socket joint.

ACL anterior cruciate ligament.

acute injury of recent onset.

adduct to move a body part toward the midline of the body.

adduction movement toward the midline of the body. Applied to the hip, it means moving the legs together or even crossing one over the other.

adhesions fibrous bands that form between tissues and organs, often following surgery. They may be thought of as internal scar tissue that connects tissues not normally connected.

ADLs activities of daily living such as walking, sitting, standing, and lifting.

aesthetic having a sense of the beautiful; pleasing to the eye and senses with regard to balance, symmetry, and grace.

agonists half of a muscle pair, the muscles that contract to perform movement.

alloy a material composed of two or more metals or a metal and a non-metal.

alpha angle a finding on an MRI that can help diagnose a cam impingement. It measures the roundness of the femoral head.

anesthesia a drug agent that causes the loss of sensation or consciousness.

anesthesiologist a medical doctor who is certified as a specialist in the administration of anesthesia.

angiography a medical imaging technique used to visualize the inside of blood vessels, arteries, veins, and the chambers of the heart.

antagonists half of a muscle pair, the muscles that relax so that the agonists can perform their movement.

antalgic gait walking with a limp because of pain.

anterior cruciate ligament a ligament in the knee that attaches from the underside of the femur (thigh bone) to the top of the tibia (shin bone). Abbreviated as ACL.

anteversion angled forward. The normal inclination of the acetabulum, approximately 20 degrees forward.

arthro Greek for "joint".

arthroplasty surgical formation or re-formation of a joint.

arthroscope a pencil-thin surgical instrument that allows the surgeon to view inside the joint by way of a miniature video system and to operate on the interior of the joint.

arthroscopist a surgeon who performs arthroscopy.

arthroscopy any surgical procedure that uses the arthroscope.

articular cartilage also known as hyaline cartilage, it is the smooth, thin layer that covers the ends of bones and protects the bones against impacting forces. The body's natural shock absorbers.

atrophy the shrinking in size of muscle tissue.

autoimmune disease when the body reacts against one of its own parts as if it were foreign. Lupus and Rheumatoid arthritis (RA) are examples of autoimmune diseases.

avascular necrosis the loss of blood supply to the hip joint, which results in the death of the bone on the ball side of the joint.

bilateral pertaining to both sides of the body.

biologics commercial products derived from biological sources used to treat or prevent disease.

biomechanics the position, posture, stance, or alignment that helps the body perform any activity most smoothly, with the least effort or strain. Efficient, good form.

BMCC bone marrow cell concentrate.

bone marrow cell concentrate (BMCC) blood and tissue withdrawn from the bone marrow, then turned into a concentrate that is injected into the body and contributes to the regenerative process.

burr down removing bone using a burr, an electrical tubular instrument with a sharp, round, bone-cutting end that spins at high speed.

bursae the fluid-containing sacs that provide cushioning around joints.

bursal sacs a more inclusive name for the bursae.

bursitis inflammation of any of the bursae.

cam a bony bump at the head/neck junction of the femur that can impinge upon and damage the labrum.

cannula a hollow tube that allows arthroscopic instruments to pass through the muscles and other tissues into the joint.

cauterize to sear with a hot instrument, especially for curative purposes.

chondral pertaining to the cartilage.

chondromalacia deterioration and softening of cartilage.

chronic persisting over a long period of time.

circumduction a circular movement at a joint. Applied to the hip, this requires that the thigh move forward, then sideways, then backward in a circular pattern.

collagen the main structural protein in connective tissue.

collateral circulation secondary vessels supplying blood to an area through indirect channels.

congenital present at birth.

continuum a continuous sequence in which adjacent elements along the continuum are not perceptibly different from one another, although the extremes are quite distinct.

contraindications things you should not do for a particular condition.

core muscles a complex series of muscles that includes everything except the arms and legs. These muscles act primarily as a dynamic stabilizer for movement, although they can also initiate movement.

cortex the outer shell of the bone.

coxa magna a larger-than-normal femoral head.

coxalgic gait walking with a limp due to hip pain.

crepitus a creaking or crackling sound or sensation when moving a joint, a muscle, or a tendon.

crossover sign a finding on an X-ray that identifies if the acetabulum is retroverted, or rotated backward, compared to normal anteversion.

CT scan computerized axial tomography. A three-dimensional X-ray that is one hundred times more sensitive than an ordinary X-ray.

debride to remove dead or damaged tissue.

deep vein thrombosis (DVT) a blood clot within a vein.

distraction gentle traction placed on a joint. Hip distraction is performed by wearing a flotation belt, then applying weights to the ankles and floating motionless while suspended in deep water.

DNA deoxyribonucleic acid is a molecule that encodes the genetic instructions used in the development and functioning of all known living organisms and many viruses.

embolism a blood clot that travels from one location to another within the body.

epidural anesthetic anesthesia given by injection in the lower back that numbs the nerves and stops the sensation of pain.

extension straightening of a joint, or as applied to the hip, reaching backward with the leg behind the body.

fascia bands of fibrous tissues throughout the body that attach, stabilize, enclose, and separate muscles, nerves, blood vessels, and organs.

femoral head the ball on the end of the femur or thigh bone.

femur the thigh bone, the largest bone in the body. The top of the femur is the ball part of the ball and socket that makes up the hip joint.

fibrocartilage the rubbery cartilage that composes the ears and the nose.

flexion bending a joint. As applied to the hip, lifting or pulling the thigh closer to the torso, or bending at the hip.

flexor a muscle whose contraction bends a limb or other part of the body.

foley catheter a thin, sterile tube inserted into the bladder to drain urine.

fracture a break or crack in a bone or cartilage.

functionability a person's ability to function within his or her personal environment.

gene a portion of a DNA molecule that serves as the basic unit of heredity. Genes control the characteristics that offspring will have by transmitting information in the DNA.

general anesthetic a combination of medicines you inhale or receive through a needle in your vein. Under this anesthesia, you should be unconscious and not feel pain during the surgery.

gluteal pertaining to the buttock muscles or the buttocks.

Golgi tendon organ a sensor imbedded deep in tendon and ligament that responds to slow stretch by lengthening the muscle. It also provides information to the brain regarding position sense.

gout a form of inflammatory arthritis that causes sudden, severe pain, swelling, and tenderness—most often in the large joint of the big toe.

growth factors naturally occurring regulatory molecules that stimulate cell and tissue function by changing their biochemical activity and cellular growth and regulating their rate of proliferation.

Health Maintenance Organization (HMO) an organization in the United States that provides comprehensive health care to enrolled individuals and families in a particular geographic area by member physicians with limited referral to outside specialists and that is financed by fixed periodic payments.

Heberden's nodes bony enlargements of the finger joints in osteoarthritis.

hip arthroplasty surgery that removes degenerated cartilage and reconstructs the hip joint using metal, plastic, or ceramic components. Also known as hip implant surgery.

hip flexor tendinitis inflammation of the tendon that attaches your hip flexor muscles to the pelvis.

hip implant surgery the technical name for surgery that removes degenerated cartilage and reconstructs the hip joint using metal, plastic, or ceramic components.

hip replacement the common name for hip implant surgery or hip arthroplasty.

hyaline cartilage synonymous with articular cartilage. The shock-absorbing surfaces on the ends of bones.

iliotibial band thick fibrous tissue that is connected from the hip down the outside of the thigh, crosses the outside of the knee and attaches to the lateral side of the tibia.

impingement the unwanted compression of soft tissue between two or more harder, unyielding structures.

implant *Noun*. That which is inserted. ***Verb***. To insert a part.

implanting inserting an implant into place.

incentive spirometer a device given to a postsurgical patient that motivates him or her to breathe deeply. Visual feedback shows the depth and strength of each breath.

internist a medical doctor certified in internal medicine.

isokinetic exercise exercise that is variable and based on the patient's strength. As the patient pushes harder, the resistance increases proportionately.

isometric exercise exercise that does not involve any movement of the joint or limb, a fixed muscular contraction.

isometrically pertaining to the use of a muscle group that contracts but doesn't cause movement.

IV intravenous fluids given to supply nutrients the body needs.

joint capsule the tough fibers and ligaments that encase the hip joint.

joint space narrowing a finding on an X-ray that is a primary indicator of osteoarthritis. It shows a loss of cartilage, hence a decrease in joint space.

KlapperVision® Dr. Klapper's verbal way of creating visualization of anatomical structures and function through the use of daily life and household analogies and metaphors.

labrum the fibrous rim that surrounds the hip joint.

ligaments strong, fibrous tissues that link bones at a joint.

ligamentum teres a fibrous band that attaches from the head of the femur to a notch deep in the acetabulum. This ligament contains within it the acetabular branch of the femoral artery.

loose bodies benign fragments inside the joint, usually of cartilage or bone.

macrotrauma abrupt tissue damage either from internal or external forces.

meniscus the shock-absorbing fibrocartilage in the knee.

microtrauma repetitive stress placed on tissues over time that results in a cumulative injury.

modality a therapeutic agent applied to a patient to reduce pain and swelling while it arouses the body's natural healing mechanisms.

MR Arthrogram a series of MRI images of a joint after injection of a contrast medium, which helps detect small abnormalities more easily than the normal MRI.

MRI (Magnetic Resonance Imaging) a diagnostic technology that uses a superconducting magnet and a computer to precisely display soft tissue and bone that is not apparent on X-ray.

muscle spindle sensors in the belly of muscles that warn muscles to contract when they are stretched so they will retain their normal length.

musculoskeletal the muscular and skeletal systems viewed as a whole.

native neck the normal shape of the femoral neck without bony defects.

necrosis death of areas of tissue or bone surrounded by healthy parts.

nerve block anesthetic numbing medication given by injection near specific nerves to eliminate pain around the hip during surgery.

neuromuscular coordination the harmonious functioning of muscles or groups of muscles in the execution of movement.

neuromuscular reeducation therapeutic exercise in which nerve signals are "retrained" and appropriate muscle movements are repeated so that movement patterns become automatic again.

NSAIDs nonsteroidal anti-inflammatory drugs.

nurturing activities that are low impact and therefore soothing to your weight-bearing joints.

orthopedist a medical doctor who is a certified specialist in treating disorders of the bones, muscles, joints, ligaments, tendons, and other parts of the musculoskeletal system.

osteopenia bone density that is lower than normal but not low enough to be classified as osteoporosis.

osteophyte a bony outgrowth associated with the degeneration of cartilage at joints.

osteoporosis a loss of calcium and bone density, usually associated with aging.

palpate to examine by the sense of touch.

passive, sustained stretch a manual technique applied by a coach, athletic trainer, or physical therapist to increase range of movement.

pathognomonic specific to one thing only.

pathologic relating to pathology.

pathological of or relating to pathology.

pathology condition produced by disease.

Patient-controlled analgesia (PCA) a device attached bedside to the IV. Preprogrammed by the doctor, it allows patients to administer preset doses of painkilling drugs directly into their own IVs at limited intervals.

PCA patient-controlled analgesia.

pelvic girdle the basin-shaped complex of bones that connects the truck and legs while it supports and balances the trunk. The pelvic girdle is made up of three bones: the ilium to the top and both sides, the ischium behind and below, and the pubis, in front.

periarticular erosions defects and crevices around the perimeter of the joint where the cartilage stops and the regular bone begins, usually seen in rheumatoid arthritis.

pharmacology the study of drugs and their origins, properties, and effects.

phonophoresis the use of ultrasound plus the addition of medicine to the water-based gel. The ultrasound thus drives the medicine through the skin into the underlying tissues.

pincer an enlarged rim of the acetabulum (socket) of the hip that can cause impingement upon and damage to the labrum.

placebo a medicine given to appease the patient but containing no true medicinal properties.

plasma the liquid portion of the blood. Plasma is derived when all the blood cells (red blood cells, white blood cells, and platelets) are separated from what is called whole blood.

platelet these cells in the blood aid in the blood-clotting process. When activated, platelet cells adhere to one another to block the flow of blood from damaged blood vessels.

platelet-rich plasma (PRP) blood plasma collected from a patient that has been enriched with platelet and re-injected into the part of the body that needs increased healing.

prehab presurgical conditioning or rehabilitation.

pre-op pre-operative, as in pre-op procedures and pre-op holding room.

proliferation rapid reproduction of a cell, part, or organism.

prophylactic protecting or defending from disease, a preventive measure or drug.

proprioception one's own perception, the sense of relative position of the parts of the body and the strength of effort used in movement.

protocol the description of the steps to be taken in a medical treatment or rehabilitation program

PRP platelet-rich plasma.

pulmonary embolism a blood clot that lodges in the lungs.

quadriceps the four muscles that run down the front of the thigh causing hip flexion and knee extension.

radiologist a medical doctor who is a certified specialist in the interpretation of X-rays, MRIs, and CT scans.

reciprocate stairs to ascend or descend stairs by placing one foot on a stair, then the opposite foot on the next stair, and to continue alternating in this manner.

regional anesthesia medicine given by injection that blocks the nerves to a specific area of the body.

rehab the conversational word for rehabilitation.

rehabilitation reconditioning of the musculoskeletal system to restore maximum function.

repeated contractions a manual physical therapy technique that begins the strengthening process for weak muscles.

replacement the act of replacing. Hip implant surgery is commonly called hip replacement surgery.

retroversion angled backward. The opposite of the normal inclination of the acetabulum, which may or may not be problematic.

revise to perform a surgery to replace or compensate for a failed implant or to correct undesirable results from a previous surgery.

revision a surgery performed to replace or compensate for a failed implant or to correct undesirable consequences from a previous surgery.

rheumatologist a medical doctor who is a certified specialist in rheumatological diseases including rheumatoid arthritis, lupus, osteoarthritis, and fibromyalgia.

rounds the common phrase for a doctor's visits to his or her patients in the hospital following surgery.

sacroiliac joint the junction where the triangular-shaped sacrum meets the pelvis.

saline solution salt water.

scaffold a structure to keep cells inside the borders of a cartilage defect and stimulate cell growth during an attempt to rejuvenate articular cartilage.

sciatica pain radiating down the sciatic nerve into the back of the thigh, the calf, and into the toes.

sclerosis an uneven hardening of the bone due to unequal weight bearing in a joint.

spinal block anesthesia injected into the fluid surrounding the spinal cord in the lower back to cause a rapid numbing effect.

spur an abnormal bone growth at the edge of joints. Also called osteophyte.

starting pain a sure sign of hip joint problem; after resting, if pain is present upon starting to move, that indicates the problem stems from the hip.

stem cells simple cells in the body that are able to develop into any one of various kinds of cells (such as blood cells, bone cells, cartilage cells, synovial cells, etc.)

stenosis narrowing of a canal or opening, often applied to a narrowing of the various openings in the vertebrae that pinch the nerves.

studies diagnositic tests such as X-rays, CT scans, MRIs, and MR Arthrogram.

subchondral beneath the cartilage.

subcutaneous beneath the skin.

synchronicity the act of being well coordinated.

synchronistic coordinated, combined.

synchronistically behaving in a synchronistic manner.

synovectomy the removal of all or a portion of the inflamed lining of a joint.

synovial fluid the lubricating fluid within the joint.

synovial lining synonymous with synovium, the lining of the joint.

synovial membrane a thin, soft, pliable layer of tissue lining the capsule of a joint. Also synonymous with synovium.

synovitis inflammation of the synovium.

synovium the lining of the hip joint.

tactile perceptible by touch, tangible.

tendinitis inflammation of a tendon.

tendons the fibrous cords of connective tissue that attach muscles to bones.

tesla the unit of measurement of magnetism, named after Nicola Tesla, a Serbian-American inventor who created the alternating current electrical system used throughout the world.

Thera-Bands latex bands used for resistance exercises.

titanium metal alloy a mixture of titanium metal and other chemical elements that is exceptionally strong and also light in weight.

vasoconstriction narrowing of the blood vessels resulting in a reduction of blood flow.

vasodilation enlargement of the blood vessels resulting in increased blood flow.

visualize a surgical term, to make visible.

X-ray electromagnetic radiation that passes through the body to create a picture of the dense tissues of the body, such as bone.

APPENDIX

The following is a list of companies with their products and services that appeared in the text.

CompletePT Pool & Land Physical Therapy

3283 Motor Avenue
Los Angeles, CA 90034
Phone: 310-845-9690
Fax: 310-845-9691
Email: info@CompletePT.com
Website: CompletePT.com

Services: Physical therapists offering pool physical therapy combined with traditional land therapy for fast, lasting recoveries. Pool sessions take place in a 92-degree, salt-water pool based on Lynda Huey's protocols. Land sessions take place in a large expansive gym. There are 18 Waterpower Workout® classes each week. One class is specifically for hips and knees.

Lynda Huey is a renowned international lecturer. She designs pools for major hospitals, clinics, and health care providers. She trains aquatic therapists from Australia, Europe, South America and the Middle East as well as from private clinics, hospitals, and universities. Lynda licenses her pool therapy protocols and electronic templates to major healthcare providers. Her techniques are available through Lynda Huey's Aquatic Rehab Online Course (AROC) at Lynda Huey.com

Huey's Athletic Network

(310) 829-5622
Fax: (310) 828-5401
Email: info@CompletePT.com
Website: www.lahuey.com
Services: Lynda Huey's Aquatic Rehab Online Course (AROC) provides Continuing Education Credits for fitness professionals and aquatic physical therapists. Visit LyndaHuey.com

Books and DVDs:
- *Heal Your Hips: How to Prevent Hip Surgery and What to Do If You Need It (Second Edition)*
- *The Complete Waterpower Workout Book*
- *Heal Your Knees: How to Prevent Knee Surgery & What to Do If You Need It*
- "Lynda Huey's Waterpower Workout" DVD.

Products:

CompletePT Flotation Belt, Waterpower Workout Tether or Tether Strap, Thermo-X shirts in both long sleeved and short sleeved styles, Neoprene Wet Shirt.

Tether holds you in the correct position for deep-water interval training. Tether strap hooks directly onto the CompletePT Belt, Wave Belt, and Aqua Trim Belt. Order tether with waist band for use with the Wet Sweat Belt and for shallow water running. The pullover Thermo-X shirt and the zip-up Neoprene Wet Shirt add a layer of warmth for exercising in cool water. Ice packs of various sizes for reducing pain and swelling.

Ace Multipurpose Wrap

Website: www.acebrand.com

Products: Hot and cold therapy products. Neoprene wraps with elastic and Velcro to hold them in place as you go about your daily life. Order the low back wrap which is also used for the hip. Order online.

Aqualogix

Website: www.aqualogixfitness.com

866-603-1156

Email: info@aqualogixfitness.com

Products: Resistance Blades–High Speed Blades and Max Resistance Blades; High Speed Resistance Bells, All-Purpose Bells, Max Resistance Bells

The blades provide smooth, effective strength training for core and lower body while the bells offer three levels of resistance for upper body and core work.

Hydro-Fit, Inc.

1328 W. 2nd Avenue

Eugene, OR 97402-4127

(800) 346-7295

Fax: (541) 484-1443

Email: hiproducts@aol.com

Web site: www.hydrofit.com

Products: Hydro-Fit Buoyancy Cuffs, Hydro-Fit Hand Buoys, Hydro-Fit Swim/Therapy Bar, Long-Sleeve Warmup Jacket

Cuffs placed on the ankles supply buoyancy during hip exercises. Hand Buoys and Swim/Therapy bar are used for support during deep-water exercise or gait training; long-sleeved jacket with mock turtle neck zips over the bathing suit adding extra warmth and 50+ UV protection.

Hydro-Tone Fitness Systems, Inc.

2468 N. Glassell St. #A

Orange, CA 92865

(800) 622-8663

(714) 998-9595 Fax: (714)998-8799

Email: hydrotone@aol.com

Web site: www.hydrotone.com Products: Hydro-Tone Boots and Bells

Products: High resistance boots to put on the feet for lower body exercises. High-resistance bells for upper body strengthening.

ABOUT THE AUTHORS

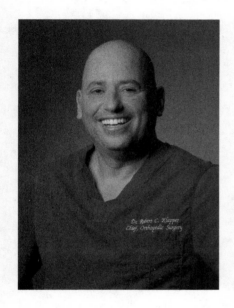

Robert C. Klapper, MD, likes to tell his patients: "My father was a carpenter and my mother was a nurse, so I was destined to become an orthopedic surgeon. The most important thing my father taught me was 'Measure twice, cut once.' It comes in handy every day I'm in the operating room."

This fits comfortably with Dr. Klapper's education and medical training (an art history degree from Columbia College, a medical degree from Columbia University's College of Physicians and Surgeons, an internship at Cedars-Sinai Medical Center, and a residency at the Hospital for Special Surgery in New York, followed by a fellowship in arthritis and implant surgery at the Kerlan-Jobe Clinic in Los Angeles), and with his bold, visionary research that has led to patents on instruments used to do complicated hip surgery. He is currently co-director of the Joint Replacement Institute at Cedars-Sinai Medical Center in Los Angeles. He has written articles for *Clinical Orthopedics and Related Research*, the *American Journal of Sports Medicine*, and other publications. He wrote chapter ten of the book *Operative Hip Arthroscopy* titled "Hip Arthroscopy without Traction." He is the host of ESPN radio's "Weekend Warrior" and the sports medicine expert on Fox Sport 1 TV.

Besides medicine, Dr. Klapper lists surfing and sculpting among his passions. He does both regularly, the sculpting in Manhattan Beach and Italy, and the surfing in Ventura and Hawaii.

Dr. Klapper can be found on Twitter @DrRobertKlapper

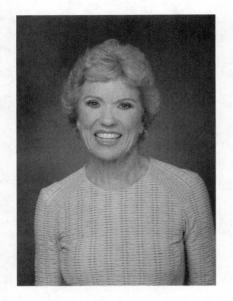

Lynda Huey, MS, starred as a sprinter at San Jose State University, earned both a bachelor's and a master's degree, coached track and field and volleyball at several universities, and wrote her autobiography, *A Running Start: An Athlete, A Woman,* before she was thirty. Her second book, *The Waterpower Workout,* resulted from her pioneering work in developing water exercises for fitness and rehabilitation of athletic injuries; and her third book, *The Complete Waterpower Workout Book,* has been the bestselling book in its field for over twenty years. She has written for most sports and aquatic rehab magazines in America and she currently writes a self-help blog at CompletePT.com/blog.

In 1999, she opened CompletePT Pool & Land Physical Therapy in Los Angeles. CompletePT has been on the list of the 100 Largest Women Owned Businesses in Los Angeles County since 2007 and has seen over 20,000 patients.

Through her fitness business, she sees many of the Hollywood elite in their home pools, and through her physical therapy business she and her staff of physical therapists treat over four hundred patients each week. She designs therapy pools and aquatic therapy protocols for major hospitals and health-care providers. She has written six books on water exercise and rehab, which are considered to be the foundation of aquatic therapy worldwide. She is a renowned international lecturer and has developed Lynda Huey's Aquatic Rehab Online Course to share her advanced techniques with students in many countries around the world.

Lynda shares the waves with Dr. Klapper as they write books. She bodyboards as he surfs. They have also written *Heal Your Knees: How to Prevent Knee Surgery & What to Do If You Need It.*

Lynda can be found on Twitter @LyndaHuey

INDEX

consulting with, 43–48, 270
examination by, 48–55, 270
pre-op visit to, 270
radiologists, 58
staff of, 46
Double Heel Lifts, 156
driving after surgery, 288
dual mobility implants, 264
dysplasia, 25, 42, 247

education classes, pre-op, 271
electronic medical files, 68
electrotherapy, 89
embolism, 278
equipment for pool program, 116–120
examination
    by doctor, 48–55, 270
    home self-exam, 41–43
exercise. *See also* land program; pool
    program; postsurgical pool program
    benefits of, 98, 202
    listening to your body, 6, 104, 106
    Negative Spiral and, 21–22, 225
    nurturing vs. abusive, 45, 82, 99,
        100–105
    reminders, 225
    reviewing your activities, 98–100
extension, 51
Extension, Prone, 13, 216
Extension with Thera-Band, 221
Extensions, 13–14, 220
extensor muscles, 20–21, 205–206, 208
Extensor Stretch, 12, 212
external rotation, 41, 51, 52
**External Rotation (pool exercises), 135,
    179, 188**
**External Rotation with Thera-Band
    (land exercise), 223**
external rotator muscles, 21, 205–206, 208

femoral head resurfacing, 263–264
femoroacetabular impingement (FAI)
    arthroscopy for, 237, 238, 239–250
    diagnosis of, 26, 44, 52–53, 69, 79
    overview, 26, 73–75
    Snibbe Stretch, 214
    symptoms of, 78
    types of, 75–78
femur, 17, 18, 26, 28–29
fibrocartilage, 31, 75
flexibility, 22, 92, 114, 140
flexion, 51, 52, 284–285
flexor muscles, 20–21, 205–206, 208,
    249–250

Flexor Stretch, 142, 182
Flies, 134–135, 178–179
**Flies Variation, External Rotation and
    Internal Rotation, 179**
flotation belts, 116, 117–118
Flutter Kicks, 146, 184
foot pumps, 265, 278
form, during exercise, 124–125
**Four-Way Hip, Three-Way Hip, 166–168,
    198**
Front Kicks, 157
Front Straddles, 155, 191
functionability, 203
functional assessment, 48
functional exercises, 230–232

gait
    abnormal, 27, 42, 62, 115, 128, 175, 202
    examination of, 42, 48
    pool program for, 115–116, 128–131,
        175–177
    treatment for, 88, 90
    visualization and, 128, 175
gene therapy, 93–95
gluteal muscle dysfunction, 249–250
Golgi tendon organs, 83, 206

Hamstring Curl, Bridge on Ball with, 227
Hamstring Curl, Standing, 230
Hamstring Stretch, 10, 12, 140, 181, 210
Hand Buoys, 116, 118
health insurance, 271–272
heart rate, measuring, 137
heat applications, 87–88
herniated disk, 64
hip distraction technique, 170–171
hip implant surgery. *See also*
    postsurgical pool program
    anesthesia for, 255, 276, 280
    benefits of, 265
    complications of, 265, 277–279, 280,
        287
    custom implant options for, 259–264
    decision for, 109, 251–252
    hospital, items to bring, 273, 274–275,
        279
    hospital procedures for, 273–277,
        280–285
    outpatient surgery, 281
    overview, 251–253
    pain management after, 279–280, 285
    postsurgical exercise guidelines for,
        173–174, 287–288, 306–312
    precautions after, 174, 283–285

preparing for, 269–273
procedure for, 255–265
recovering from, 280–290, 291
types of, 253–254
hip joint. *See also* cartilage
    common conditions of, 19, 22–33
    healthy, 17–19, 61
hip muscles. *See* muscles
hip replacement surgery, 253
history, physical, 35–40, 45, 47
home environment, after surgery, 271, 279
home self-examination, 41–43
hyaline cartilage, 18–19. *See also* cartilage
Hydro-Fit Buoyancy Cuffs, 116, 119
Hydro-Fit Hand Buoys, 116, 118
Hydro-Fit Shirt, 120
Hydro-Fit Swim/Therapy Bar, 118–119
Hydro-Fit Wave Belt, 116
hydrostatic pressure, 112, 293, 307
Hydro-Tone Boots, 116, 119, 194

ice applications, 86–88, 280, 292, 297
Iliotibial Band (ITB) Stretch, 213
impact exercises, 151–162, 189–193
impingement. *See* femoroacetabular
    impingement
implant surgery. *See* hip implant surgery
incentive spirometers, 280
infections, 47, 273
insurance benefits, 271–272
internal rotation, 51–52, 284–285
**Internal Rotation (pool exercises), 135,
    179, 188**
**Internal Rotation with Thera-Band
    (land exercise), 224**
internal rotator muscles, 21, 23, 205–206,
    208
Interval Training, Deep-Water, 136–139, 180
**Interval Training, Shallow-Water,
    160–162, 193**
isometric exercise, 208

joint. *See* hip joint
joint capsule, 18, 21–22, 50, 214
joint space narrowing, 61

kicking exercises, 144–150, 155, 157–158
    postsurgical, 183–188, 192
Knee Swivels, 8, 166, 197
Knee to Chest Stretch, 11, 211
knees, 27, 42–43, 50

labral tears
    arthroscopy for, 238, 239, 240, 241,